THE COPING
CAPACITY
*On the Nature
of Being Mortal*

THE COPING CAPACITY

On the Nature of Being Mortal

by
Avery D. Weisman, M.D.

Copyright © 1984 by Human Sciences Press, Inc.
72 Fifth Avenue, New York, New York 10011

Printed in the United States of America
123456789

Library of Congress Cataloging in Publication Data
Weisman, Avery D.
  The coping capacity.

  Bibliography: p.
  Includes index.
  1. Adjustment (Psychology) 2. Death—Psychological
aspects. 3. Cancer—Patients—Psychology. 4. Terminally
ill—Psychology. I. Title.
BF335.W415 1984   155.9'37   83-26659
ISBN 0-89885-206-4

Greatness is a conspiracy,
Genius is an accident,
Wisdom is an achievement,
But survival is a conundrum.
ADW

CONTENTS

PREFACE   *xi*

CHAPTER 1.

The Case for Self-Instruction   *1*
Abiding questions and ordinary problems   2
Self-instruction and coping well enough   4
The case for enlightened skepticism   7
Autonomy and authority   9

CHAPTER 2.

Cancer Mortality and Other Expectable Problems   *13*
Cancer: disease, myth and mortality   *15*
Other expectable problems   *19*
  Sickness serious enough to matter   *21*
  Calamity and catastrophe   *22*
  Deterioration and decline   *23*
  Uprooting and disruption   *24*
  Dysphoria and deviance   *25*
  Incapacity and disability   *26*
  Demoralization and disenfranchisement   *27*
  Death and deathliness   *28*
Three basic metaproblems   *30*

CHAPTER 3.
Common Coping Strategies 31
What is a metaproblem? 33
Caveats about coping 34
Common coping strategies used by you and me 36
Coping strategy 1. Seek information; get guidance 37
Coping strategy 2. Share concern; find consolation 38
Coping strategy 3. Laugh it off; change emotional tone 40
Coping strategy 4. Forget it happened; put it out of
your mind 42
Coping strategy 5. Keep busy; distract yourself 44
Coping strategy 6. Confront the issue; act accordingly 45
Coping strategy 7. Redefine; take a more sanguine
view 47
Coping strategy 8. Resign yourself; make the best of
what can't be changed 49
Coping strategy 9. Do something, anything, perhaps
exceeding good judgment 50
Coping strategy 10. Review alternatives; examine
consequences 52
Coping strategy 11. Get away from it all; find an escape,
somehow 54
Coping strategy 12. Conform, comply; do what is
expected or advised 55
Coping strategy 13. Blame or shame someone, something 57
Coping strategy 14. Give vent; feel emotional release 59
Coping strategy 15. Deny as much as possible 60

CHAPTER 4.
Between Vulnerability and Morale 63
Precepts for good coping 64
Vulnerability and what it means 66

Four existential plights   70
  Annihilation   70
  Alienation   72
  Endangerment   73
  Denial   74
Illusion and the unlived life   76
Appropriate death and the reality of illusion   80
Angst and vulnerability   82
Primary morale   83

CHAPTER 5.

Coping, Countercoping, and Psychotherapy

Coping, Countercoping, and Psychotherapy 85
Cancer and psychotherapy   85
Countercoping and its counterparts   89
Tasks and techniques of countercoping   92
Psychotherapy: the unobtrusive intervention   94
Encounter, empathy, and failure   102
The therapist's consolation   108

CHAPTER 6.

The Ten-speed Life Cycle

The Ten-speed Life Cycle   112
What makes the life cycle circular?   115
Ten subcycles to cope with   116
  Chronological uniformity amid change   117
  Developmental interaction   118
  Physical well-being and health   119
  Psychosocial adaptation   121
  Psychosexual fulfillment   122
  Racial, ethnic, cultural, and tribal *et ceteras* 123
  Ideological affiliations   126
  Personal and mental distinction   127

Politico-economic deployment 130
Thanatologic realization 132

CHAPTER 7.

The Survival of the Dodo 134

Intermediate strategies 136
What did the Dodo in? 138
Coping with coexistence 142
Does old age make sense? 145
Omega values and vulnerability 146
    Exemption from the work ethic 147
    Freedom for individuality 148
    Undistracted self-instruction 149
    Short-term goals and long-term motivation 149
    Uncertainty and solitude 150
    Passionate sublimation 151
    Forgiving nature and tolerating mortification 153
    Vicarious participation 154
    Communication between generations 155
    Triumph in death 156

BIBLIOGRAPHY 158

INDEX 163

PREFACE

Man is the measure of what is human, and he is also the measurer.

But how shall man be measured, since most of our thinking is done through images, metaphors, analogies, and words that for the most part fortify and perpetuate our prejudices.

There are no natural, unequivocal units for measuring the level of humanity that mankind reaches or fails to reach. In my opinion, humanity is measured in several ways, ranging from our skill in coping well to our achievement in surviving according to the best standards of which we are capable.

One indispensable measure of humanity is our capacity to cope humanely with problems that present themselves, generation after generation. Because problems are apt to persist, recur, or only seem resolvable, the task of coping needs the support of courage and morale.

We rue the brevity of life. Frustration, discouragement, and very meager rewards await even energetic and courageous efforts. In everyday life we mostly struggle in solitude, unable to grapple with the obscure dilemmas that perplex existence. Paradoxes proliferate; absolutes are elusive, yet we presuppose them and could not survive without the illusion that some generalities are truth and some truths are general. We have no gods who seem willing to take our case and plead our cause, whatever that is. Consequently, we are thrown back on our puny resources, seeking to develop ways and means, methods and strategies, for coping, quelling, and living significantly. Why we do so is itself a problem to reflect on.

No one who thinks about the perils of existence will fail to realize that among all the problems and deplorable conditions surrounding us, the most basic issue is how to cope with so many assaults on survival. Furthermore, we survive on many planes, each one of which decides what the others mean because they are all necessary for significant survival.

Challenges to existence go beyond the obvious ones of war, famine, disease, poverty, natural catastrophes, and now the brooding presence of nuclear incineration. There are daily threats to humanity, not just existence. We note quiet erosions of character, impoverishment of spirit, decay of morale, fall in self-esteem, abandonment of purpose, a general invasion of vulnerability.

Survival alone has little or no significance. The requirements of humanity insist on survival with competence and a purpose, whatever they may be. But we also are faced with shortcomings and vulnerability that are only satirized by appealing to lofty, pious aims beyond our capacity. Promises of vague rewards sometime, somewhere may seduce millions but largely cause more pain and mortification than inspiration.

Within the past few decades, this terrified century has witnessed the growth of a curious discipline, concerned with all kinds of death-related phenomena. To be sure, next to love and sex man is always very interested in death and ways to postpone or deny it. Love and sex are much more welcome, but the field of thanatology has permeated almost every aspect of human thought and behavior. In my opinion its major contribution has been to encourage more candid examination of the facts of death and our presuppositions about it. Death is an essential part of humanity, although we have tended to push it to the periphery, out on the far edges of existence, as if it applied only to the very aged or to "other people."

Death will not stay in the shadows, because more people—facing the threats to humanity on a large scale or even in our neighborhoods—recognize that we do not confront death in the aggregate, from disease or war, but inexorable personal death.

In this book, I propose to look at how we very ordinary folks cope and fail to cope with a variety of regularly occurring threats to our integrity and survival, which I term *expectable problems*. Learning to cope with premonitions of that final scene, the moment of inescapable extinction, provides us with a series of coping strategies that enable us to deal with a thousand other earlier problems and dilemmas.

I have begun by examining the ways in which cancer patients come to terms with their disease and its psychosocial ramifications. Cancer is a contemporary scourge that, despite the disclaimers of medicine and research foundations, has come to acquire a metaphorical and mythic significance because it is the protoype of fatal illness and therefore the symbol of death and deathliness.

Other diseases may have a far more ominous outlook. And for certain types of cancer the chances of cure are solid enough to encourage hope for recovery. Not so with other kinds of cancer, which almost at the moment of diagnosis are beyond treatment.

In this book I am primarily concerned with cancer mortality, which, besides its medical meaning, has strong symbolic significance. It symbolizes a threatening and dreadful fate, largely consisting of such expectable problems as are embodied in fears of invalidism, intractable pain, untold suffering, humiliation, and everything else that can undermine a significant existence. My concern with cancer, moreover, is to demonstrate that how we cope with a prototypical disease permeates the strategies we use to cope with other threats to survival. Problems that baffle us with respect to cancer mortality also baffle us when these problems simply impose a threat, without an accompanying medical disease.

In a general sense cancer mortality is also a myth, and myths are models of the way we personalize the indifferent forces that threaten us. Myths are mirrors in which our own reflection is caught. Myths are under no obligation to be logical, reasonable, or to respect facts. Consequently, cancer mortality is mythical because it challenges significant survival and typifies much of which we are most afraid. Actual statistics about cancer mortality are somewhat beside the point. Cancer mortality as a myth represents the enemy, more hostile than death itself.

At its very cruelest, cancer the myth is only a prototype of many problems that represent the human predicament. These concerns perplex and defeat even staunch and capable efforts to cope and to prevent their occurrence. Of course, no one person falls victim to every devastating problem; that would simply be too outrageous. However, these cancer-like problems that obstruct us from a more harmonious existence happen so frequently and profusely that we can readily, soberly, bitterly call them expectable.

Despite what must seem a very gloomy attitude toward mankind and its abiding problems, I believe that we can and do develop very effective and versatile coping strategies. Courage and morale are inseparable; each strengthens the other, and despite fears or cowardice, we can enhance the likelihood of dealing well enough with problems as they present themselves.

The journey toward limbo really should be conducted by a new John Bunyan who is absolutely sure of his destination and can confidently safeguard his charges. But times have changed; no one can pretend to absolute understanding and foreknowledge. I am a very ordinary person who has observed, pondered, and tried to understand how other ordinary mortals confront and deal with their own vulnerability to expectable problems. Furthermore, I have witnessed prodigious efforts and accomplishments as a result of coping with what seemed like overwhelming problems. These are not academic matters but existential brinksmanship with the most serious obstacles people are likely to face, either their own death and disability or what is often more painful, the intractable suffering and death of someone deeply loved.

It is fitting, therefore, that an ordinary person undertake to describe these mundane yet singular events. To draw back out of a genuine dread of deficiency would violate the principle of self-instruction and the goal of coping well enough. It is easy to become demoralized, but by lowering expectations and adopting other strategies one can regenerate courage, redefine problems, and replenish one's own morale. I offer readers that same encouragement and hope.

I do not limit this book to familiar discussions about psychiatric and psychoanalytic topics. Instead I try to deal with paraclinical issues, which are authentic sources of suffering rarely written about in the psychiatric literature. A jungle of jargon, combined with highly specialized polemics, makes finding one's way through to a clearing extremely difficult and unrewarding.

Everyone must be an existentialist of sorts, depending on their perception and appreciation of existence. And where psychology and psychiatry end, philosophy takes up the slack. But philosophy hardly goes very far, despite its pretensions to world views. That we are all joined together means little more than being shackled by our ignorance, inertia, and special interests.

Existentialism is a misnomer for the highly personal, private, idiosyncratic attitude we adopt toward our own life and death dilemmas. What really counts most is not our attitude toward speculative issues but how we deal and cope with everyday concerns and mundane issues that threaten us, block progress, and show us up.

No less than you, I must learn to cope well enough with one problem in order to be ready for the next, expectable or not. I cannot, therefore, put my own feelings aside and hide behind a mask of pseudo-objectivity. Every person is objective but only in his fashion. Man is the creature that copes with contingencies. In doing so he pretends to be less vulnerable than is true.

Problems undergo transitions at different ages and stages of various life cycles. Ordinarily, description of life cycles begins at the beginning and then postulates a series of phases that are presumed to be equally relevant for practically everyone. We know how even careful physical anthropologists have fooled themselves and others in tracing the development of humanoids as well as horses. There is something about the life cycle that not only seduces people into making grand generalizations but leads to self-deception on an even grander scale, much as a child given a set of paints and a lot of paper will certainly cover it all.

Efforts to understand how human beings get to be as human and inhuman as they are are pilgrimages that founder, because they lead into quagmires of causality and development that in retrospect seem rather pretentious and pathetic. Most "begin from the beginning" accounts of development concentrate on early times—when a child is born, grows up, turns into an adult, procreates, and then, somewhere midway, changes. Documentation becomes sketchy, surmises expand, and interest wanes. Old age and death-related events are still off at a distance, largely ignored, but pointed out.

My interest in the impact and ramifications of life-threatening illnesses and behavior prompts me to consider the strategies of coping with pervasive problems from the perspective of old age, concern about death, and the singular values we seek.

If coping with contingencies is mankind's primary way to find significant survival, then an examination of old age and its concerns should be informative, especially about those values that turn out in the long run to be most important and effective. This should be quite enough, without the luxury or indulgence of looking for a deeper significance or "meaning." After all, maturity must be good for something, besides waiting for inevitable devaluation and obsolescence.

I have tried to be tentative and adumbrative, not dogmatic. Most people like to make the same claim, and like most people I have only the courage of my prejudices and presuppositions. Nevertheless, good coping requires us to challenge what has worked before, even if it means defying one's own bias. For instance, I believe that exceptions to a rule evoke a refined rule, without necessarily refuting or rationalizing it into a false consistency. When dealing with the elusive, tantalizing criteria for the worth of man the measurer, it may just as well be done by scrutinizing old age and the perspectives of death.

Just as a sense of reality senses what reality testing supposedly tests, a sense of responsibility is a response to a variety of directives and prohibitions. Collectively, these become the cultural standards for what is expected of us. Thus, the standards are readily exchanged for what we do, fail to do, consider worth doing, and think we do when we don't.

These imperatives, quiet and loud, are the unspoken, vivid, tacit criteria that measure the worth of man, and that man uses for everyone else. Nevertheless, every discipline, whether called a science, art, or trade, tries to understand its own special version of ambiguity and uncertainty. One such discipline is psychoanalysis, which explores man's motives, conflicts, and deceptions. From my viewpoint, psychoanalysis has great potential for studying how people explore their own motives and vulnerabilities. And this has been a principal preoccupation and profession for me. However, I am here mainly concerned with how ordinary people, not in psychoanalysis, cope with everyday problems, not with the intricacies of defenses and conflicts. Our common fate is coping with coexistence, and this, surely, is a problem for humanity at large and for humanistic disciplines of all kinds.

I shall deal with weighty matters, but I intend not to make these chapters topheavy with theory and jargon that only specialists have familiarity with. I will often refer to death and other deadly matters, since we can all expect to die sometime, but to speak of the devil is not a formal invitation. We can approach the problems of limbo and coping with relative ease, knowing that we are learning how to deal with difficulties with composure and competence.

I am most comfortable when dealing with middle-level abstractions that grasp facts of experience with one hand, while reaching for more comprehensive theories with the other. The journey toward limbo can take many directions; it uses conveyances of all kinds and certainly travels at different speeds. I believe, urge, and demonstrate that coming to terms with inevitability and being able to cope well enough to survive significantly are not only feasible, practical, and constructive, but in the end, liberating. This is the only true freedom.

ADW

CHAPTER 1

THE CASE FOR SELF-INSTRUCTION

As this century winds down to an inglorious and foreboding conclusion, those of us who are unlikely to witness much of the next must now pause a bit and ponder what our brief presence was all about.

Here we stand, still mystified by the arch of heavens, insecure, vaguely disturbed, puzzling over our precarious place between the oceans. This is the only moment we shall have or, to be precise, truly know anything about. And before the onrushing tide of years engulfs this time and place, there are questions that roil up over and over, just as with generations long vanished. What justifies being alive in the first place? How do we manage with a never-ending supply of distressing problems? Why do we cling to existence if it is that much trouble? Of all these problems, which are the truly serious issues and which are merely fraudulent annoyances? How do we measure and apply standards to our efforts? What constitutes failure, how shall we best cope, which problems are expectable? And so on.

ABIDING QUESTIONS AND ORDINARY PROBLEMS

An abiding question is, of course, one without a permanent answer that satisfies everyone. Nevertheless, it is a question that bestirs us to pursue principles and to question traditional policies and ingrained beliefs. Is coping an art, a science, a skill that can be learned like a language, or is it simply an accident of birth and fortune? Considering the risks and resentment that most creative or rebellious deviants incite, how independent or autonomous dare we become? Perhaps we are better off doing what we are told instead of seeking information and confronting problems as they arise. Whatever we do, we can be sure that we are adopting one or another coping strategy, and each strategy is a tiny fragment of the totality that I call the journey toward limbo.

About one thing we can be very sure: to ask what life means is an utterly meaningless question, not even an abiding question. Where is the index or context of reference that would enable us to answer such questions? Until and unless we get beyond and outside life itself and find a perspective for evaluating values, life itself has no meaning whatsoever. What the pseudoquestion ostensibly means is what values are worth pursuing. But lacking an outside vantage point, this question can only be echoed, not answered. The echo consists of tautologies and analogies that leave the problem just as enigmatic as ever. We do not ask what life means, therefore, but we can seek the perspective that tells us what reference points to use in establishing the value of what we do.

Every generation chants its own precepts, proclaims its mythology as clearly established, and offers its manifestos as truths. Generations have their favorite generalizations; ours is no exception. At best, generalities are true only for some people under special circumstances and are useful under even more limited conditions. Scientific truths get that way by making limited conditions quite explicit, instead of sweeping away doubts and misgivings with mere decibels.

No one has the inherent right to speak for everyone else. This democratic ideal is a good example of a generalization with many limitations, external and internal. We grant that no one has the wisdom, knowledge, and compassion to know what is best with absolute certainty. But there are many who reverse this generalization, declaring that because we have power, we also have certainty and with it, the wisdom, knowledge, and compassion to use it effectively.

On a smaller scale, there are many who profess to have the resources to feed our hunger for leadership and to tell us what to believe in, think about, be, or buy. Their merchandise comes in many packages for instant consumption. Their strategies are oratory, rhetoric, appeals to bias, and browbeating.

The only alternatives to being led and misled by forceful or benign propaganda are submission, resignation, and opposition. But these strategies do not neutralize the effect; they reinforce the efforts of those who dominate by deed or precept. How difficult it is to cultivate and instruct ourselves in the mysteries of a perspective that judges but does not promise too much in the direction of requiring complete understanding or in answering abiding questions that have not been raised.

This century has raised questions that challenge existence itself. Are long perspectives really available? Or are we too fragile to defy efforts to force submissive agreement? Yes, longer viewpoints are accessible. Even now, history is being made, evolution is going on, and glaciers of events are drifting relentlessly, but there are other events that the sweep of human history glides over. These are the problems of ordinary people. In contending with them, we sometimes reach a comfortable resolution; often they defeat our best efforts. What problems can these be? How do we cope with them? Which guideline is relevant?

There are guidelines for almost every proposed action—except that more often than not they are obsolete, irrelevant, misleading, and propagated only to reaffirm an established loyalty.

Basically, we are alone, just one in a crowd of survivors, seeking the best way of managing poorly understood problems. Certainly only a few people concern themselves with the forces that got us here and will take us away. This moment is passing, and we still look for a purpose in having been here to undergo the trouble and travail that seem to be an inevitable heritage. Since no authority we rely on seems to respond, we cope as best we are able, given the obstacles impeding the journey from day to day. Obviously, total mastery is an illusion, and so perhaps is the idea of total submission.

SELF-INSTRUCTION AND COPING WELL ENOUGH

Our modest aim is learning how to cope well enough for practical purposes, and all good coping is practical without necessarily being ideal, propitious, heroic, original, or transcendent.

Reality is certainly practical, interlaced as it is with fears and expectations encased in mystery. Coping well enough must deal with whatever reality presents, regardless of how it is construed. Coping requires a preliminary and provisional anticipation of feasible consequences. This effort makes certain actions more promising than others, and not, therefore, just a matter of luck.

But after all, reality of even the sturdiest kind is partially composed of fabrication colored by wishes, habits, bias, and factual fragments. Facts are only low-level theories that most people we know tend to agree about; proof consists largely of what we already believe and would like to document further. As a result, most disputes and their settlement simply falsify or silence the beliefs of those who do not agree with us.

Good coping does not stay at this primitive level. It depends on improving what we perceive and how we interpret facts, gathering more information and correcting our performance in managing problems. Unfortunately, in some instances good coping is simply equivalent to reiterating the popular beliefs so convincingly that there is never a good reason for deviation. In such instances, "coping" is seldom a significant issue.

Coping well enough requires a measure of autonomy, as well as self-conscious questioning. Otherwise, it is a mechanical, reflex obedience to commands, in which case we might as well relegate everything to our masters. If not, then the capacity to deviate successfully in response to an assessment of consequences and alternatives *for us* is what I mean by *self-instruction*.

Coping is a skill, not a science. It uses a mixture of facts and fabrications, deals with whatever information is available as well as what can be only conjectured about. Because we see dimly, it must be followed by whatever our best judgment—and there is no other—decides.

If we are to survive unharmed and unendangered, emerging problems need to be coped with. Most of us are not concerned with the big history of wars, nations, politics, and the achievements or failures of first-magnitude people. We are simply concerned with *our* history and prospects, gnawing on our own particular bone, as it were, and finding it buried when and where we want it. Our history puts our signature on what we do and endure. It also contributes to what we stand for, or call truth and fiction.

Coping well enough is an attainable skill acquired by self-instruction, with perhaps a little help from others. But its goal is never actually completed, contrary to a dog's task of burying a bone and digging it up again. Whatever happens, we can be sure only that reality presents us with an ample package of ambiguity, uncertainty, ambivalence, and anxiety.

Problems do change. They will remain somewhat the same in their basics, but different enough to call for different solutions. The range of self-instruction is limitless—the world is the tutor. It has very little to do with education or inculcation of belief. Its precepts are beacons that may distort or disguise, but the good coper learns to self-instruct by differentiating between the real and the respectable.

We learn very little from famous personages whose lives and deeds comprise much of history. As ordinary people, very little of what we say or do anywhere will be noted or long remembered; it is unlikely to influence multitudes. Luckily, that is an irrelevant consideration for everyday purposes. It is the mundane but extraordinary event that calls on our efforts to cope with its problems and consequences. Santayana's famous aphorism about remembering the past lest we repeat it is not only quoted out of context but is singularly disingenuous. When we remember the past, we are as likely to repeat it as to modify our behavior and correct mistakes. Problems and occasions are seldom precisely the same, but we are apt to respond as if they were. We readily and self-righteously make similar mistakes, over and over.

Self-instruction will use the past, but in revising, correcting, and perfecting strategies for dealing with newer problems, we must learn how to forget the past. This is, of course, difficult to do; sometimes it is necessary to realize that tradition and established authority are based on the presumptions of very fallible people who improvised and fabricated just as we do. Good copers seek to liberate themselves by questioning the unquestionable, tolerating deviance, even looking for hidden truths in long-established errors. Self-instruction cultivates uncertainty in order to use it, since there are no universal truths that can be fully relied on.

In the detritus of history we can find almost any lesson we want. We learn and learn to avoid in order to cope better. But who is qualified to be our instructor and mentor? Only those who recognize the preeminence of self-instruction. As a rule, the world insists on its own convenience and conformity; we choose not to comply at our own risk. Innovation is often bitterly discouraged unless it substantiates what mentors would have us believe. Custom, therefore, is another word that means to conform and agree with precedent; it also recommends coping with problems in the same old ways, regardless of whether such efforts worked well or not.

The repetition compulsion, itself a tenacious tenet of psychoanalysis, asserts that we repeat behavior over and over, irrespective of consequences. As a result, we find ourselves again and again in similar predicaments, doing what custom decrees and we hardly ever dispute.

Nevertheless, manners change, problems differ, and transitions alter cases. Each day we are more alike than different simply because my identity is me; I am destined to sustain myself, like it or not. Either my world changes and I remain the same, or I change while my world reproaches me.

Heraclitus notwithstanding, you *can* step in a river more than once, and may even slip and fall. Human predicaments are more complicated than stepping into a river or learning to swim. The very old often are accused of being too fixed, too soft, too atrophic, too little, or too much of many traits and characteristics. Surely, experience and self-instruction must provide them with some reliable strategies to protect them in old age. The answer is that with the passage of years and the transitions of problems, certain older people do remain fixed and immobile, acting only on the basis of older situations without accounting for newer revisions. The ability to change with the times means the capacity to redefine new problems as different from older prejudices. Of course, almost everyone will claim having an open mind and being up-to-date, even if they shake their heads and deplore deviant opinions and embarrassing facts. Voltaire's memorable proclamation about being willing to defend to the death an opinion he disagrees with is hard to accept. Most of us would not defend even what we agree with, lest we get involved. We might quickly glance around and forsake private opinion, coping with threats by adopting an attitude and strategy that counsels conformity and compliance. We are not heroes.

THE CASE FOR ENLIGHTENED SKEPTICISM

The proper place for enlightened skepticism is midway between abject cynicism and bedazzled conformity. It is a frame of mind that both protects us against the inroads of dogma and offers an escape from dismal negativism. More important, the enlightened skeptic disputes and finds reconciliation with ideas and practices that are merely sanctioned and popular. Many people are our unwitting mentors, even the anonymous "they" who disapprove any traces of deviance in our behavior.

Formal education has its deep and abiding values, but self-instruction often must combat the axioms and anathemas of entrenched knowledge. How, for example, are bigots formed? Education and social class by themselves provide only a respectable rationalization for the vulgarity and violence hiding beneath social prejudices. No amount of class work or reading lists will chip away at group hatreds and suspicions. Through self-instruction we learn that bigotry is bad for us as well as for the others whom we categorically despise, but it is a lonely enterprise. Its purpose is to discover a finite number of expectable problems lurking amid different situations and then to call on different strategies with versatility.

That we are fallible and faulty scarcely needs emphasis. Diverse philosophers agree that the ideal of education is to equip us to be on our own, but they stipulate that being on our own should carry additional values and obligations besides creature comfort. The ideal of psychotherapy is also that of being on our own. Whether the therapeutic aim is symptom relief or self-actualization, having a broader range of independent action compatible with civilized society is axiomatic. But it should be combined with a self-conscious significance for being alive.

Self-instruction combines the aims of education and psychotherapy with much self-help. In struggling along, we carry the impediments of the past, including its errors and misconceptions, into the present, with its own problems and perplexing ambiguities. When we learn to cope better, spontaneity and skill gradually permit us to relinquish the past and to retain only those fragments that are still useful. Self-instruction is an unending task. It strives to discriminate between the price and value of what is offered as choices. The ideal education, seldom reached, also provides a wider set of choices as well as different styles of assessing which choices are worthwhile. Analogously, psychotherapy gets rid of whatever impedes choice and seeks to improve conduct in the search for advantageous values.

We learn a little from the past but must divest ourselves of much that is burdensome. In a less certain sense, the future is also there to offer self-instruction. Socrates professed to believe that an unexamined life is not worth living. While this generalization seems to refer only to a philosophical turn of mind, another meaning is that Socrates recommended self-instruction in the consequences of what we do and strive for. Self-exploration seeks to understand better what we are and might be but are not. It does away, we hope, with self-deception. Nevertheless, many unfortunate people pervert self-exploration and confuse it with perpetual self-excoriation. Either they think that everyone else has or is something better, or that they have failed in whatever task confronted them. Guilt is not a good guide, nor is shame the test of personal significance.

We do learn from consequences, and in doing so, we prepare for the future. Preconceptions are not prescriptions, but unfortunately, the most entrenched assumption is recognized last. Insofar as self-instruction is education, our course is an open cirriculum.

AUTONOMY AND AUTHORITY

There is no other struggle so old, so exasperating, as that between autonomy and authority. This is the reason for seeking a reconciliation through self-instruction. The conflict takes many forms, and I shall not attempt to describe how different types of discipline and power have been set up to enforce one side or another. In everyday affairs we little people also struggle to reach a balance between personal freedom and protective, potentially coercive authority.

Except for very polarized societies, it is sometimes difficult to tell the difference between autonomy and authority. What is called autonomy may be only a more intangible form of authority that is no less coercive, while commonly agreed upon authority, protested against and even reviled, actually may serve the interests of the individuals covered by its acts. The balance between autonomy and authority is not necessarily one of politics. When I am ill, my autonomy is impaired. I submit myself to the authority of disease, which has mighty coercive powers, and to its representatives, the medical professions, and its institutions. My autonomy is further compromised when I become a hospital inpatient. I obey rules, take medicine, agree to procedures, and hope to recover without much impairment or delay. When I am discharged, medical authority is relinquished; my autonomy is regained. How I will then use autonomy is up to me; perhaps this is the key meaning of autonomy: having to decide what to do with the freedom one experiences. Authority in its best sense facilitates creative use of autonomy. Self-instruction, also in its best sense, decides what kind of authority is best able to protect the freedom to cope well.

Brave words about freedom and coping with the future, but we need to be reminded that except for instances of extreme authoritarian control or of meaningless freedom without power, we are all pilgrims. Not only do we not know how we got here, but we are not at all sure where we are going. It is always wise to ask ourselves, "What am I doing here?" Inevitably we continue, but our steps may waver between autonomy and authority as destinations vary. We may even retrace our steps and find that we are back at the beginning, without any better understanding of how we got there. A pilgrim is not a prisoner condemned to plodding in circles or digging holes only to fill them up again. A pilgrim is one among many who wonder what unspecified authority has set forth so many paths.

One of the lessons learned from the future is that autonomy is an acquired taste, not a natural state of mankind. Many people, including hordes of pilgrims, are anything but autonomous and have no taste whatsoever for autonomy's rewards. Authority is an established reference point that can be very consoling, reliable, and stabilizing, and not all authority is automatically bad. Neither can exist without the other. Authority needs autonomous people to subject themselves and self-instruct themselves in coping strategies.

Few of us are pioneers or prophets. We need guidance, not just in precepts but in learning how to avoid and overcome obstacles. Benevolent authority, which is not dictatorship in the cause of someone else's powerful autonomy, is useful and imperative. Without it, autonomy is absurd. Not all institutions are invidious, nor are men of power necessarily callous and cruel. We are governed, as our leaders and institutions are, by ideas, relationships, symbols, and intangible meanings and rules that defy definition.

To summarize: our unique pilgrimage in this everyday world is destined to find a congenial sense of reality in which we create a productive balance between autonomy and authority. We want to be free to choose the kind of authority that governs us. This means freedom to act and revise our beliefs, and in doing so, promote the cause of self-exploration. Compromise is an obligation, but compromise does not mean resignation. Coping is always the aim, even if our strategies oscillate wickedly between extremes. We can learn to be active in this sense, passive in another sense; we are coercive and compliant, aggressive and submissive, dedicated to both altruism and self-interest, committed to science but practicing a kind of sorcery, and so on.

Although we are immersed in the past, autonomy can rescue us by anticipating and advocating a congenial authority. We anticipate consequences, thus changing the past and breaking out of ancient molds. Sometimes we find that the ancient molds have only reconstituted themselves in the guise of discovery.

As pilgrims, we may, therefore, retrace our steps and find that a prolonged pathway leads back to where it started. Similarly, entrenched authority may be defied; by using autonomy in ways that do not invite disaster, we discover that freedom has brought us full circle. In a real sense this is not a discouraging redundancy but perhaps a tribute to having learned to cope well enough to master problems that got in the way. Each generation learns to survive on its own terms. We can fall victim to a variety of prototypical diseases and forsake autonomy. Cancer is very coercive in this respect. It persuades us about our vulnerability but insists that we cope as well as possible, without polarizing ourselves between a useless freedom to die or a disappointing authority that promises more than can be delivered.

Coping well enough owes its effectiveness to *both* autonomy and authority. I walk erect only because eons of development and a succession of imponderable genetic contingencies have ordered it that way. I grasp a pencil, for example, and at that instant share the act with my arboreal ancestors swinging through trees. Similarly, in human behavior, our self-instruction does not arise out of a vacuum but depends on a tradition that imposes limits and guidance.

Man is not a rational animal, except when nothing much is at stake. Otherwise, he is a rationalizing beast seeking to save his skin on the best terms negotiable. In this respect, philosophy and ethics are uncertain guides. There is much authority surrounding mankind, but much autonomy can be mustered to control and come to terms with disenfranchising elements.

The case for self-instruction depends on the belief that coping well enough is the hallmark of autonomy and that capitulation is not a universal remedy for discontent. Even that rationalizing beast called man needs periodic infusions of self-esteem, enthusiasm, and morale in order to realize and make real the self-conscious side of humanity. *Otherwise,* efforts to educate, explore, and survive are just a charade that disguises our impotence. *Otherwise,* my advocacy of self-instruction would be a hypocritical counterfeit. *Otherwise,* exhortations about freedom tantalize without fulfilling.

Morale is not a rational sentiment; it need not be. Courage is in the same plight, because we must concede our limitations, deceptions, and difficulties. Morale and courage may require the risk of setting forth on missions without a purpose.

Nevertheless, self-instruction is not altogether an illusion. *Otherwise,* our destiny would be no more enlightening than the unceasing slothfulness of coral clinging to a rock beneath the sea. Autonomy uses authority, and authority is molded by autonomy. There is no panacea, no ambrosia to satisfy all hungers, and no absolute truths. But there are absolute falsehoods and many partial truths. As pilgrims we shall find better ways to test the reality confronting us, and in doing so, being tested by that reality, we construct newer versions of what is real and worth coping with.

CHAPTER 2

CANCER MORTALITY AND OTHER EXPECTABLE PROBLEMS

We live within such narrow boundaries of health and disease, safety and disaster, normality and deviance, that to survive at all, as well as we do, is almost a miracle. That we can also thrive under inauspicious circumstances is even more incredible. Nevertheless, despite overwhelming threats and actualities, here we are.

None of us is exempt from multiple dangers that regularly confront us from all sides. Although the truly wretched have vastly more problems, the very privileged—as we are who, for instance, have access to education, affluence, and health—are not spared private catastrophes.

The potential for injury, insult, invalidism, devastating illness, and destructive behavior lurks in everyone, despite being steeped in self-protective and self-righteous illusions. Perhaps it is just as well that we minimize these various risks because our frailty cannot be denied.

If we turn to the rewards and benefits of survival, certain puzzles and paradoxes emerge. If, for example, to survive simply means to avoid various dangers indefinitely, how is it that sufferings of all sorts are not enough to dissuade most of us that there is no point in clinging further to a life that has such dubious value?

The rationality for survival is unpersuasive. Mere endurance is itself a vacuous prize. But rational suicide is equally objectionable, and for all but a few people it is a perversion of reason. True enough, many courageous people forfeited their precious lives unwillingly when faced with the alternative of a death camp. But it is paradoxical that under circumstances of misery, pain, discontent, and repeated disasters, so few of our fellow men and women opt for suicide. An even greater puzzle is why mankind can tolerate almost limitless anguish, only for the questionable privilege of suffering awhile longer.

Injury, illness, inanition, suicide, homicide, and senectitude are common causes of death. But these are only the end points of problems that preceded and predisposed its victims. Survival can be as rational or irrational as suicide, except that rationality has little to do with either. There is no truly acceptable reason for continuing to live, except that we want to. Ultimately, however, the drive to survive yields to the disposition to die, just as sleep overcomes wakefulness. Despite wide differences in our pace, the corridors of time narrow for everyone.

I need not further document nor support the contention that nature's bounty largely consists of more problems than we can possibly solve with meager equipment and desultory incentives. My vision of man as pilgrim seeking an up-to-date version of salvation and significance must now, in these closing years of the century, confront another image, the spectacle of man as eternal refugee from evil. Nothing is too preposterous, and our vulnerability is wide open to new antisurvival forces.

I need to be forgiven a musty academic aroma when, in an effort to bring down a profusion of problems to a comprehensible finite number, I refer to *modalities of misfortune*. These constitute extended but far from infinite dreads that we call *expectable problems*. These modalities are multifaceted. What I call "expectable" is not necessarily certain or even predictable. It is only because no one is spared totally that their occurrence imposes much concern, terror, anxiety about existence itself. Consequently, such problems and modalities are thoroughly expectable. If not, then look at the daily newspaper and find evidence of death, disease, disasters, demoralizations of all kinds abundant enough to generate dread.

CANCER: DISEASE, MYTH, AND MORTALITY

Today's archetypal modality of misfortune, expectable problem, and antisurvival force is *cancer.* Not only is it common (in this country second only to cardio- and cerebrovascular diseases as a cause of death), but it creates and foments much terror. "Tell me, doctor, could this be cancer?"

I must distinguish cancer the disease from cancer the myth and cancer mortality. Full discussion of cancer the disease belongs to other places, other authors. There are, however, several hundred diseases that fulfill criteria for neoplasia and are called cancers. Only a few are common enough to be looked for and warned against in everyday life. Cancer the disease comprises the statistics for cancer mortality, but the myths about cancer and the cancer metaphor that derives from its mortality go beyond the problem of cancer treatment.

Cancer the myth is a widely disseminated product of facts and fears, consternation and fantasy, that agonizes and frightens millions. Despite considerable efforts to allay such fears, countless people are sure that to be diagnosed as having cancer is but a prelude to dying of cancer. Physicians themselves often deny the diagnosis of cancer and delay consulting other doctors. The myth of cancer permeates even our language and idioms—"Mr. President, there is a cancer growing . . ." To speak of cancer directly, instead of referring to a "tumor" or a "growth," is almost an obscenity, without the accompanying chuckle. Cancer the myth is more than a public health problem that can be controlled by education. It is a symbol of pain, exhaustion, helplessness, and dehumanization.

Cancer mortality has become a metaphor transcending bound-

15

aries of disease. Insofar as cancer is considered an evil, death is its object lesson. The metaphor and myth extend throughout human discourse and seem to evoke universal dread of antisurvival forces.

According to legend, the Four Horsemen of the Apocalypse were War, Pestilence, Famine, and Death. Obviously, so few horsemen could not possibly represent all the threats and dreads that abound; there are just too many for a single metaphor—a cavalry would not be enough. Nevertheless, war, pestilence, famine, and death are amply represented in the mythology of cancer mortality. And we shrink, terrified, from this specter.

Much of what is reported in newspapers and magazines about cancer sounds like dispatches from a war zone. And much more than body counts or tactical engagements are involved. Cancer is the enemy incarnate, and medical research pits itself against battalions of antisurvival cells, as in some modern-day Armageddon. While the number of dead is hard to conceal, typical reports emphasize the positive and imply an imminent though modest breakthrough. Research results are often bruited in the same way that minor skirmishes are magnified into major victories.

Although cancer is a serious, frequent disease, it is by no means inevitably fatal. The myth and metaphor do not allow for cures and remissions. Consequently, a recent survey showed that most people believe that cancer is less common than it actually is, and that treatment is less effective than it can be. Fear of cancer amounts to a social hypochondriasis, not unlike dread of devastation related to war.

Cancer is also interpreted as a pestilence or plague, capable of sweeping through families, societies, neighborhoods, going from generation to generation. The prospect of becoming a cancer "victim" conjures up visions of wasting away, starvation, vomiting, intestinal obstruction, disgust for food, and so on—all of which corresponds to cancer as cause of famine. The dread of intractable pain and agony means famine from within, because the unfortunate patient literally starves amid suffering of all kinds.

Cancer the myth only feeds the metaphor of cancer mortality.

However, the metaphor is linked to much older, but equally sinister afflictions that once carried a stigma, taboo, and mandatory sentence of death. Victims were ostracized once their disease became known, as if in the hypocrisy of mankind, evil concealed is more tolerable.

These older afflictions with sinister significance include prototypical diseases such as leprosy, plague, tuberculosis, and syphilis. Fortunately, practically every case can now be cured, although their names will still evoke a shudder of dread. Cancer is now by itself among the prototypical diseases for which no cure is thought to exist, so evil are its consequences. Prejudice pours into the vacuum of ignorance, and as a result, victims are blamed and shamed. In effect, victims become presumed victimizers and therefore are enemies to be shunned and segregated.

Why? One reason is that a victim of a prototypical disease reminds everyone of how vulnerable and helpless we are. Another reason is the very common tendency to blame the victim, either for an ugly deed we might well commit ourselves or for having a flaw or secret that deserves punishment in the shape of misfortune. For both reasons, the hapless, blameworthy victim or perpetrator is sent away, out of sight, to an asylum, prison, segregated compound—just anywhere where harm will not befall us.

The cancer victim also is seen as the victimizer who causes or transmits evil. While it is probably too strong an indictment to claim that cancer the metaphor criminalizes the disease, there is no lack of prejudice. Victims are, implicitly, put into another social class, and like most fearful victims, they are treated with a mixed attitude of deference and disdain. Certain cancer symptoms seem to be greeted with an air of disgust and distaste not found with other illnesses. Bigotry and prejudice about cancer victims and victimization assume different forms in various social groups. Some former patients, for example, report that they were asked to use a segregated toilet or towel or washbasin when they returned to work. On a higher level of prejudice, a skilled computer scientist asked, rhetorically, "What would you do, Dr. Weisman, if you were a personnel manager and had two people, equally qualified, applying for the same job? Wouldn't you find some reason to give the edge to a healthier person who hadn't had cancer?'' Compassion often fights a losing battle against antipathy.

There is a popular but thoroughly unproved theory that ascribes cancer to the inability to express hostility or to manage grief adequately. This is a very old theory of psychosomatic disorder that marshals many anecdotes, simply because in our society hostility is supposed to be restrained. Furthermore, we lack precise understanding of what constitutes adequate management of grief. The public at large usually avoids or shuns anyone viewed as harboring too much resentment or anger, as if such people are dangerous to be around. Those who are grief-stricken and very depressed are also troublesome; they tend to transmit sadness and dejection, contaminating the atmosphere with discouragement and despair. Perhaps there is folk wisdom in the customs that isolate bereaved family members until they get over the acute phase of mourning. Maybe such customs are intended to benefit the nonbereaved people just as much as, if not more than, those who are very sad, depressed, and dejected.

Older prototypical diseases had their own mythology of contagion and corruption. For example, in biblical times, leprosy was considered a sign of being accursed, and its victims were doomed to forfeit everything valuable and become beggars. Syphilis was for a long time known to be associated with sexual contact, but until recent times it also symbolized gross immorality and, to use a Victorian term, excess venery.

Although some writers, such as Sontag, found that tuberculosis had a quietly romantic penumbra, most people used the epithet consumption, which meant a highly lethal disease brought on by extreme poverty, lack of sanitation, and bad heredity. It was a disease of lower social classes.

My purpose in associating cancer with other legendary diseases, and calling all of them "prototypical" is that their metaphorical or psychosocial significance was much more inexorably evil and hopeless than the facts justified. I must make an exception for plague, which decimated Europe and then practically disappeared. Occasional cases do turn up but without the taint that it once had, possibly because cures are possible. A curable disease is not a curse, nor is it wholly evil. But if an illness is both prevalent and very serious, if not inevitably fatal, it becomes prototypical for a variety of social ills, which is a metaphor in itself. As a result, the disease draws to itself a number of other intractable problems and dreaded outcomes from sources outside the province of medicine. Cancer mortality, therefore, symbolizes any tragic, dreaded fate that may be a consequence of being alive.

Other expectable problems are linked with cancer mortality because we feel utterly unable to cope with them, and as a result we are exposed to antisurvival forces that, like so many demons, pervade existence and strike us down.

OTHER EXPECTABLE PROBLEMS

Expectable problems are not exceptional problems but only seem that way. Their frequency is often underestimated by some, overestimated by others. For example, death from cancer is a less obtrusive preoccupation among actual cancer patients than it is with many other, relatively healthy people who are quick to fear cancer whenever they have an unusual ache, pain, or bump.

Because the range of human problems, even expectable problems, always exceeds its boundaries, the following list cannot pretend to completeness, however abstract I try to be. My purpose is served, however, if the reader just looks over the list and sees if he or she ever feared any of these problems. What would you do if you were faced with such a problem? How might you cope with a dilemma that seemed uncopable?

Here are a few "other expectable problems" besides that of cancer mortality:

(1) Sickness serious enough to matter
(2) Calamity and catastrophe
(3) Deterioration and decline

(4) Uprooting and disruption
(5) Dysphoria and deviance
(6) Incapacity and disability
(7) Demoralization and disenfranchisement
(8) Death and deathliness

If all these problems seem to be the same, they are not, although they may overlap. Moreover, problems in general tend to resemble each other, but people with those problems are exceedingly unique. Therefore, nothing I subsequently state can be true for everyone, but much will be true for someone, somewhere sometime—and in greater numbers than suspected. No one is an exception, although we might in our ignorance believe them improbable.

Belief that we are exempt comes from not having yet fallen victim to a prototypical expectable problem. However, we do tend to believe that the world *as we know it* is under some sort of reasonable control. We also believe that we might have something to do with tipping the scales in our favor through good behavior, good luck, or good heredity. Certain very optimistic people even maintain that justice and fairness play a part in the world's operation, contrary to every indication.

These sentiments are difficult to relinquish; they might even come in handy one day, if any of the foregoing misfortunes occur. Nevertheless, for a few minutes, I ask that these beliefs about justice and exemption be set aside. Let us imagine, not unreasonably, that all of us are as vulnerable as anyone else and not exempt for any reason. Let us also "pretend" that no one or no force is really looking after us or offering protection. Nor is there much we can do on our own, except to the extent that we can cope within modest limits.

The foregoing list can be discovered in many areas of life, each providing its own set of calamities and sources of consternation. Problems starting in one area may swiftly slide into another, and then another, until a pyramid of disasters accumulates.

Here is an example. A man is out of work and has a financial problem. However, he has unemployment insurance, and until this runs out, he can be worried but capable of sustaining himself and his family. Then he is called back to work again and thus avoids the potential for calamity, catastrophe, and demoralization.

Another man, also unemployed, is not called back. He becomes alarmed, discouraged, demoralized, feels unworthy, believes himself unemployable, and soon sees his life to be one of failure, complete and unrelenting. It is an enormous catastrophe.

The difference between these two unemployed men is no greater than if they had two forms of the same cancer: namely, periodic or indigenous unemployment, a disease in its own right. In the first case, the cancer is localized and dealt with precisely and appropriately. The man copes well enough on unemployment checks, and in due time he is returned to work and undergoes a remission of unemployment. When relapse occurs again is left undecided; maybe he will work through to retirement without further layoffs.

In the second case, unemployment is the prelude to a disease course that ends in destruction of self-esteem and morale. The man's way of life is destroyed; he is invalided in an economic and spiritual sense. Throughout his illness, which admittedly was not unexpected, he might have called on coping strategies that turned out to be ineffective, at least in preventing spread of problems to other areas of his life. He is as good as dead.

But each expectable problem on my list does have special characteristics and deserves separate consideration.

Sickness serious enough to matter

Good health is the prerequisite for every other satisfaction. Some people do seem to tolerate frailty and even serious illness better than others do, demonstrating a bounce and benevolence that surprises everyone who comes near. Good health requires a sturdy constitution, coupled with reasonable guidelines and a temperament for seeking and using good information and help. It also requires much luck, and of course, diligent, persistent coping in order to maintain healthy standards and high morale.

Good health is usually taken for granted until it is lost or taken away. Since physicians cure only a few diseases, prevent some others, and relieve a certain amount of discomfort until an illness goes away, sicknesses serious enough to matter are maladies that are neither mild nor self-limited. Unless a patient recovers on his own, serious sickness will find many tests, much advice, and doubtful help.

I find it curious that people will buy sweepstakes tickets in the hope that, despite long odds, their number will come up for the big score. At the same time, however, they continue to drink and smoke excessively, gaining weight, and trust that, despite short odds, their number will not come up for that even bigger score. The latter is another example of feeling exempt, despite risk, while the sweepstakes gamble shows traces of a trust that somehow they will be rewarded. Seemingly harmless risks are undertaken readily, as if luck were under control by someone, somehow, in our favor. Bad luck is usually considered just that, until we realize that sickness serious enough to matter may be at least partially brought about by our negligence and sense of exemption from this expectable problem. Taking a chance is a policy as well as a coping strategy that suspends good judgment.

At the other extreme of risk taking are those unfortunate enough to blame themselves for misfortune. Their strategy is playing it safe, being very cautious and circumspect but also seeking to appease the gods who control the fate of man. If their life goes well, it is, for them, an omen of impending bad luck. But when sickness serious enough to matter develops, they do not blame bad luck but themselves. Whatever they do is wrong, simply because being alive is a no-win situation.

Calamity and catastrophe

Calamities and catastrophes are like being struck by lightning: improbable but usually fatal. Being mugged or raped on our city streets is becoming much more probable, and although fatalities do follow, many unfortunate victims are so violated in body and spirit by the event that it haunts them for years afterward. The very frequency of attack, or similar unprovoked abuse, violates everything most people think belongs to an orderly world. Whatever violates, let alone destroys an attitude toward life, property, person, and morale, can inflict permanent damage. Mundane antisurvival forces conspire in ways that are as devastating as earthquakes, which at least are shared with the community.

The external form of a damaging and calamitous event may not always be felonious. We may, for example, be a little supercilious when a mother weeps because her child did not get into a fashionable school. A minor traffic altercation presents little cause for alarm. Nevertheless, minor incidents are not always trivial. Everyone is vulnerable in special ways. Years later, a rejected application or a humiliating argument in traffic may still rankle and cause lasting, though quiet shame. It is especially unfortunate when others are later blamed for being at fault.

One can define a problem and deal with it, but one cannot pick or choose which problem to have. Certain problems are courted, if not encouraged. A man who proclaims himself a loser and a failure usually begins by tolerating disappointment poorly. Then he anticipates further difficulties and may perhaps act in ways that invite refusal, rudeness, defeat. People defeat themselves in many ways, ranging from lack of self-confidence to a sense that everyone else is unworthy and so deserving of nothing but unspecified revenge. Actions and attitudes have a way of disclosing themselves, subtly creating antagonism, and if carried over to job and personal relations, they may precipitate and prolong repeated failure. In our society failure and uncertainty are grievous faults. They amount to calamity.

Deterioration and decline

Self-respect is a tiny tyranny, and low self-esteem is a harsh, unyielding taskmaster that undermines diligent, admirable efforts and almost certainly turns success into failure.

Deterioration and decline are slower versions of calamity and catastrophe; they are just as painful and destructive as abrupt breakdowns. Simple but repeated disappointments, frustrated efforts that fail over and over are preambles to gradual erosion of body and spirit. Willy Loman has become a folk antihero, a ghost with a shoeshine, that all men dread.

There must be a reason why psychiatrists are asked, "Is this normal?" Patients are deeply and quietly concerned about poor memory, awkwardness, ease of fatigue, bad sleep, disturbing dreams, and a hundred other complaints that incite a fear of incipient deterioration.

Reassurances to the contrary, a time comes when the "normality" of deterioration and decline is no longer tenable. An expectable problem presents itself, requiring a degree of coping effectiveness that bodily and mental integrity may not be up to. We may be asked to run when it is difficult to walk or climb stairs.

Two common examples of deterioration and decline are progressive invalidism, which means physical helplessness; and senility, a combination of grossly impaired psychological and physiological well-being. Roles and relationships also will suffer, and the gap between what was and what has become is wide and painful. It is not quite a pun to note that when people become invalids, they also become "invalid" as autonomous individuals. In fact, they are remnants, leftovers, tattered strangers who only look familiar but no longer have a functional and contemporary purpose in the world and among people closest to them.

Uprooting and disruption

Other expectable problems arise when, after a seemingly simple move from an old neighborhood, certain people feel estranged and depressed. Familiar landmarks and clues for a reality that can be depended on are replaced by alien expectations.

Considering how often the American public moves about, leaving one area and taking up residence in another scarcely seem unusual or pathogenic. Friendships are lost, people lose touch, entire families go years without meeting.

Moreover, it is often a sign of growing up when a young adult moves away from family and old friends and becomes autonomous in another city. But moving away voluntarily is different from forcible change or deprivation. This is true uprooting, the mildest symptom of which is nostalgia and loneliness.

In order to cope effectively, we need either environmental stability or personal strength to withstand changes of an unwelcome kind. The difference between a retiree moving south and a refugee moving toward an uncertain sanctuary is enough to demonstrate that uprooting and disruption come about when our environmental base is disturbed and we have little to say and do about it.

Uprooting and disruption also can occur without geographical change but with intense internal transformation. There is no more profound example than in mourning and bereavement. Death imposes a calamity in some instances, a disruption for others. The world is empty. Familiar relationships seem strange and strained. Reality testing itself has lost an important ally. It is therefore wise for an acutely bereaved person not to make any more changes than are absolutely required. Stability is mandatory if, in time, a tenacious past is to be let go. Such existential uprooting is prevented by gradualism and surrender of what is no longer relevant.

Dysphoria and deviance

Dysphoria is a technical term used by professionals to denote a bad feeling. It is synonymous with distress, anguish, severe discomfort, or any of a number of unacceptable emotions that we would like to dispel. Unless dysphoria is dispelled, painful emotion is likely to take over one's life, undercutting constructive efforts and setting up a kind of internal dictatorship over what one does and feels. Hence, composure is a virtue that keeps dysphoria in check. Conversely, dysphoria is likely to be accompanied by deviance in behavior. It is also a sign of problems not coped with.

The deviance I speak of is not that of antisocial behavior but rather that of difficult, strained, tenuous relationships with other people who are put off by lack of composure, defensiveness, argumentative manners, and frequent complaints about mistreatment. Just as often, the victim of dysphoria spread wide into distress realizes that he or she also has deviated from acceptable norms. "I should not act this way, but I can't help flying off the handle." "I can't pull myself together." "People must think I'm putting this on, but it's beyond my control!"

Much of what is considered normal depends on conformity and control. And much of what is deviant and dysphoric is primarily distressing because it violates normality and seems beyond control. Yet dysphoria and deviance are expectable problems because no one is so assured and self-contained that every event is met serenely and effectively. Symptoms of such existential deviance are not only alien but alienating.

Not every instance, nor most examples of dysphoric deviance are found among borderline personalities (whatever that rubric means). A cancer patient who isolates himself, broods incessantly, answers monosyllabically to solicitous questions about his health, grunts instead of being grateful, is not a law-breaker, nor even a marginal personality, but an emotional deviant. His aggrieved silence is alienating, as if he is reproachful. Silence can be a sign of composure, but in this case, silence is an ironic travesty of self-containment. Dysphoria and deviance have created an estrangement that provokes anger and circular resentment in those caring for and about him. Note, however, that despite a dysphoric rift, no overt feelings are expressed.

The sharpest, most alienating dysphoria known to those who suffer is that of intractable pain. Pain is not only a powerful persuader but an antisurvival force. It is so exquisitely internal that even the most sympathetic onlooker feels helpless to intervene, and to the victim the personal agony is beyond the reassurance of shared experience. Pain erodes self-esteem, limits choice, and destroys autonomy. Those who find pain somewhat praiseworthy because mild pain alerts us to overstimulation and exhaustion would not find prolonged pain very redemptive.

Incapacity and Disability

We are all incapacitated to some degree but by no means disabled. For example, few of us are capable of writing a great sonnet, composing a symphony, or building a space rocket. These shortcoming are incapacities that impose no handicap. To be disabled is more authentically personal, since it is the groundwork for demoralization. A helpless person might hope for a reprieve or other positive change. A hopeless person may not even be helpless but self-defeating.

Fear of incapacity and disability haunts the healthy, even at moments of triumph and during a lifetime of effectiveness. Hence, it is an expectable and harassing problem: to anticipate a sudden reversal of fortune or a blow of fate that condemns a person to hopeless, helpless dependence on others, assuming that someone is available. If chronic failures help bring about their calamities, then those who are more successful may still dread having everything taken away and being reduced to utter disability and dependence.

Anticipation of *copelessness* is a modality of misfortune that undermines the prospect of being alive and thriving. Physical incapacity is bad enough, but when coupled with a conviction that there is no use dealing with the consequences of disability, the only recourse is suicide.

Demoralization and disenfranchisement

Demoralization is an entropy of hope, effort, and aspiration. Everything seems depleted and barren. Expectable problems no longer can be distinguished from one another because misfortunes have fused into an amorphous mass of misery. Coping is an alien notion, and hoping for any positive change is a forbidden sentiment.

Some psychiatrists maintain that it is demoralization that makes the difference in sending people to seek psychotherapy. As a rule, few people voluntarily consult psychiatrists. The grossly psychotic or antisocial are largely compelled to be evaluated. But the person who is unduly agitated, afraid, depressed, or perplexed will postpone counseling with a professional until they are on the ropes, nearing a knockout, feeling helpless and certainly exhausted.

I believe that it requires a generous measure of honesty and courage to admit to oneself that help is needed, to seek out and to cooperate in the rigors of a psychotherapeutic venture. For some people, demoralization prevents them from *wanting* help, because hopelessness and futility are too strong. Such people feel only doom and defeat; anything more positive is a mockery. Their motto is "Nothing can be done."

Disenfranchisement means that a person is totally engrossed in defeat and depletion. Such an individual feels no right to protest, to register a belief, to claim any privilege beyond that of being miserable. "It is too late, doctor, I cannot change." It is a careful psychotherapist who does not fall into the pit and resign himself to sharing failure. When anyone, therapist or client, is abjectly resigned to whatever might come up, then he is close to feeling disenfranchised, because protest is always possible. A good counselor knows that if there is not total tragedy, there is room for improvement, largely because the seeming calamity or disability or demoralization can be coped with.

When a client or patient feels total demoralization, then psychotherapy is almost useless, especially if that person perpetuates his sense of disenfranchisement. The therapist will be fended off, just because he symbolizes a trace of hope. The result is a stand-off; the therapist is rebuffed and the patient is confirmed in negativity.

Death and deathliness

The proposition that mortality means an obligation or duty to die is hardly original. Nor is the idea that having potential for death and dying is part of the human predicament. However, it is not usually recognized that underneath most human problems, including the expectable modalities of misfortune on my list, is a wellspring of doubt and concern about death or survival. The dilemmas of deathly fears and beliefs are sustained by vulnerability and dread of despair.

Deathliness is not deadliness. A bullet is deadly; so is a poison. But more intangible threats, such as those I have called expectable problems, contain deathly elements. It is the difference between a deadly assault and a deathly foreshadowing of doom. Incessant guilt, boundless shame, repeated self-abasement, disenfranchised surrender to intimidating specters—all are examples of deathliness that damages the spirit of being alive and thriving.

There is a familiar, even "basic," paradox in man's recognition that all men are mortal and his inability to accept the reality of personal extinction. In short, it is said, he cannot imagine himself dead without also being an observer of a dead body that looks like him.

What this paradox amounts to is our insistence on being at the cognitive center of any world we can imagine, even a nonworld after our death. However, it is wholly possible to overcome the paradox by eradicating deathliness from the idea of dying and then accepting our inevitable demise. Organic death becomes the uncertain pact we have with the future. Only the date is left blank on our death certificate.

Meanwhile, every misfortune draws on dread and risks of death and deathliness. Consequently, every culture or society decrees that death is a time for mourning, at least (or at the most), a token of having known an evil that the rest of the clan fears. Our deepest expectable problem, therefore, comes down to a confrontation of good and evil.

Another version of the good-evil dilemma is that which asks about the values worth seeking. What pays off in the end? Conformity, compliance with expectations, or individual strivings against the stream of conventionality? Pleasure, hedonism, or contemplation?

Is cancer mortality good or evil? Are sickness serious enough to matter and the other expectable problems good or evil?

Cancer mortality, serious sickness, and other expectable misfortunes are problems because they *interfere* with living on as high a level of thriving as possible. In themselves they are evil only if we have illusions about living immune to suffering or indefinitely postponing death. Death can solve almost as many problems as it creates; it is not an unmitigated evil. Although there is probably much good in curing serious illness and thwarting death for a while longer, there is much evil in pretending that death can be put off, again and again, until a person practically lives forever. Credos that refuse to recognize mortality and that insist on tying death and deathliness together assume that to die is an evil thing, in which one is either a victim or a victimizer.

Fear of dying is the result of questioning the value of whatever we attempt to do during the course of healthy living and coping with misfortunes. Expectable problems are not insoluble. It is only the prospect of not reaching an idealized solution that induces dread and failure, demoralization and despair. We can cope, and learn to cope better. We cannot eliminate problems and certainly cannot eradicate death. Such is not a value we strive for.

THREE BASIC METAPROBLEMS

Exemption from death is an illusion that is as pernicious and misleading as that of absolute cancer mortality. Even in a deadly, deathly world, we can cope well enough with the expectable problems—though, of course, we prefer not to. Nevertheless, the threat of not being alive need generate no more fear than necessary, if we sustain confidence in the values and meaning we find and pursue and struggle for.

The journey toward limbo may be mitigated in its difficulties if deathliness is neutralized by accepting our finitude. Larger human issues, such as war, disease, poverty, famine, and other abasements, are likely to be around for a long time, much longer than our span. Meanwhile, truth is our only consolation.

If it is true that expectable problems and modalities of misfortune are perpetuated and draw on basic dreads of death and deathliness, we can still cope well enough with the consequences. Among these consequences are three main metaproblems:

(1) search for meaning;
(2) maintenance of morale;
(3) negotiation with death.

These three metaproblems will be our guide when in subsequent chapters we consider how best to cope, as well as what we can best cope with and for.

COMMON
COPING STRATEGIES

There are so many authorities, self-anointed and authentic, who are ready and even eager to offer advice, wisdom, and instruction for solving the world's problems that it hardly seems necessary to undertake self-instruction for coping better. It would be far easier to yield, do what we are told, follow clear guidelines, and go along with the crowd.

Whether in the long run such acquiescence—itself a coping strategy—is more effective than strenuous self-exploration or practicing a variety of other coping strategies I do not know. It depends on the importance and severity of the problem. There are certainly circumstances in which resignation and compliance seem more prudent. But not all problems can be resolved in this way. Conformity has its value but also its price: forfeiting autonomy and elevating authority to an absolute level.

In this chapter I intend to examine a number of common coping strategies which most people, including you and me, tend to call on when faced with difficult problems.

Despite our vaunted pride in individuality, most of us are

uniquely gullible to the quick-fix promises of fad and nostrum. We are always on the alert for self-improvements, whether to lose weight effortlessly or to attain spiritual transcendence and enlightenment by listening to a few cassettes. There are proponents of remedies for every imaginable foible and fault. People come forward with cash and credulity in direct proportion to the unlikelihood of perfectibility. It should not be surprising, therefore, that someone, someplace, has a sure-fire method for fulfilling every wish and resolving sticky problems. These methods appeal to self-help but actually exploit our tendency to do what we are told.

The pleasant patina of easy solutions for hard problems covers a very sad fact: the human enterprise, which means at bare minimum staying alive and coping barely well enough, has more potential for tragedy than for redemption and triumph. Even as we warm ourselves at the fire of temporary surcease and modest success, danger and disaster stand on the periphery of our camp.

I cannot caution often enough how precariously our efforts hang together. A slight miscalculation, an unforeseen barrier, a small deviation from routine, and, through no fault, it is all over, except for a small newspaper item.

Why study and practice coping? The basic reason is as self-evident as the dictum that it is better to know how to swim than to drown. Although it is tempting to let others prescribe coping behavior for us, this decision to forfeit choice is itself a strategy. We accept the reality of oblivion without endorsement. But this plain fact is hardly reason for forfeiting individuality and autonomy, nor does it cancel out the challenge of coping better than we do.

If there is any purpose in being alive or in searching for meaning, it must include the double goal of coping better and tolerating distress. Given our uncertainty about any world beyond this one, better coping may promote more effective survival by bringing problems down to human size for ordinary people to manage. We may be exhorted and persuaded to follow grandiose visions, but nothing can be done unless we develop skill in dealing with the practical problems of everyday life.

Coping well is a skill, and part of this skill is an ability to

identify the problems we are good at and know most about. A sculptor copes better with a block of marble than with a cornfield needing to be harvested. A plumber can clean out a stopped-up drain pipe, but he probably would be unable to cope with a broken leg.

Coping is the language of existence. It has a history, grammar, etymology, and skilled practitioners. There are special technical languages and art forms that call on various tactics. The vocabulary of coping is both simple and complex, but there are rules, traditions, conventions, and customs that mark out the acceptable forms in which problems present themselves for coping.

Like any other language, coping begins in infancy; a child learns from its elders, scholarly niceties are largely irrelevant, and fluency is more effective than being grammatically correct. Consider, for example, how languages evolve and change in accordance with society and its needs. Each generation will cope with different problems, or at least traces of previous problems, cast in new forms. In our present postindustrial society, many unemployed or underemployed people are in transition from problems once considered solved by assembly lines and strong unions—to another age, parented by computers and automation, and a set of issues with which most people are unable to cope. As a result, older problems are now irrelevant but far from solved.

WHAT IS A METAPROBLEM?

A metaproblem is what remains after more manifest problems have become irrelevant or temporarily resolved. I have already cited the *search for meaning, maintenance of morale*, and *negotiation with death* as three basic metaproblems.

There are undoubtedly other metaproblems that extend from generation to generation. Although obsolescence changes the form of various problems and potential misfortunes, solutions have a way of washing aside, revealing how temporary, redundant, and incorrect they were. Obscure multitudes have died on forgotten battlefields because of problems now obsolete and by our standards inconsequential. Yet nations went to war and people underwent unspeakable cruelties, because victors coped in one way and victims surrendered in another. Both gave unswerving loyalty, faith, and, of course, ample corpses. These multitudes wanted to survive but were induced to accept as their own some transient problem of power or prestige that purportedly had no other solution than to put the population's life on the line.

Yes, coping is a language, but problems are expressed in different idioms and accents through the ages. Cope one must, but it may mean death for a cause. These causes are only temporary, without the enduring threads of metaproblems winding their way from one period to the next. Sacrifice is only one strategy. The problem that calls for such forfeiture may be only a token of current fashion, propaganda, or salesmanship. Nevertheless, such problems awaken life-and-death loyalty because they promise to answer metaproblems like our pursuit of meaning, morale, and postponed mortality.

CAVEATS ABOUT COPING

My viewpoint is that because problems change, at least in outward form, from one era to the next, coping strategies also change. Under certain conditions, active strategies are more effective than those counseling passive preparation. Sometimes rebellion seems appropriate; at other times a more traditional, conservative set of ritualistic procedures is practical. There are tillers, entrepeneurs, professionals, and lots of others. Flexibility in using and perfecting one set of strategies or another depends on knowing what one does best and could do better.

Problems will not go away, nor can they be avoided entirely. Perfectibility is an illusion but so is the untenable delusion that coping is a futile enterprise.

The most cogent caveat about coping is that it is something that everyone does, but few people do it very well. Because much depends on the initiative of the self, good coping requires self-exploration, self-instruction, self-correction, self-rehearsal, and self-assessed consequences. At the center, man is the measure of all things, including himself.

Coping strategies do not come clearly labeled, with instructions, ready to be put together and used effectively for well-defined purposes. In the previous chapter I described a series of expectable problems, including cancer mortality, with which anyone would have trouble coping. In ordinary life, however, we could not survive unless many problems could be coped with effectively and solved. This can only mean that in our particular way we confront issues and match designated problems with prospective tactics that are likely to succeed. Such endeavors go on automatically, without much forethought, and become habitual.

In order to understand how we cope, I warn that better solutions depend on defining the problem to be coped with clearly. For example, if someone tells me he has a problem with his car, I must ask what problem that is. Was he in an accident? Do the brakes work? Is he unable to meet monthly payments? Each unspecified problem calls for a more or less corresponding strategy, which would be inappropriate if it were used for other problems with the car. Obvious as this caveat may seem, many people rigidly refuse to deviate from traditional methods in coping with newer problems. How best to cope with problems at work necessitates careful appraisal of the specifics of problems, with whom they occur, and under what circumstances, together with an inner try-out or rehearsal of what one might do or refrain from doing.

In what follows I will try to describe some fifteen distinct strategies, along with their antitheses, that people like us commonly use. But few strategies are very explicit. They are quite permeable, easy to blend with others, and not at all exclusive. Although most generations of strategies are drawn from a community's vision of what constitutes valuable and successful acts and aspirations, few strategies are directives or prohibitions for ethical, moral behavior.

Perhaps the most important caveat about these strategies is that they will, at best, only indicate what people *tend* to do and do effectively. I will be unable to tell which strategy is substantively better than the next. Every strategy and its antithesis can be perfectly valid and effective, given the right time, place, problem, and person to carry them out.

Before proceeding further, it is worth making a distinction between coping and defending. This is by no means a purely academic problem because *to be defensive* is a phrase that belongs to popular epithets, while to say, "I'm coping as well as possible," deserves at least self-serving praise.

Coping is a strategic effort to master a problem, overcome an obstacle, answer a question, dissipate a dilemma—anything that impedes our progress. According to Haan's astute interpretation, coping deals with an open system of options, while defending is essentially a closed system. Although there is no good reason why coping and defending cannot go on simultaneously, defending fends off and coping tends to resolve a problem. When one defends, the primary aim is to do away with dysphoria. The purpose of coping is to clarify and contend with a problem as adeptly as possible. Defending tends to turn a problem into a nonproblem, with which one is then, understandably, comfortable. Coping is a form of negotiating a series of obstacles, some of which are due to self-deception. It is positive in approach; defending is negative.

COMMON COPING STRATEGIES USED BY YOU AND ME

1. Seek information; get guidance.
2. Share concern; find consolation.
3. Laugh it off; change emotional tone.
4. Forget it happened; put it out of your mind.
5. Keep busy; distract yourself.
6. Confront the issue; act accordingly.
7. Redefine; take a more sanguine view.
8. Resign yourself; make the best of what can't be changed.
9. Do something, anything, perhaps exceeding good judgment.

10. Review alternatives; examine consequences.
11. Get away from it all; find an escape, somehow.
12. Conform, comply; do what is expected or advised.
13. Blame or shame someone, something.
14. Give vent; feel emotional release.
15. Deny as much as possible.

Coping strategy 1.
Seek information; get guidance

Perhaps the most commonly *reported* strategy people use in dealing with any problem is to get some information and guidance about what to do.

Information itself comes in many shapes, sizes, grades, and quality. Some information is trustworthy, but much is one-sided advice, opinion, or prejudice. Few people really know how to tell the difference and may not even care. As I have already indicated, the quick fix exactly fits many impatient people eager to improve themselves or to get rid of an annoying dilemma without drastically expending much effort.

In the field of medicine the favored coping strategy these days is to ask questions and get guidance about illness and treatment. But the authoritarian image of the physician does not easily dissipate. Too many patients are still apologetic about asking questions, afraid of seeming stupid, and incurring the contempt of their doctors. Unfortunately, there are still physicians who confuse giving information with being directive. And as everyone knows, it is easy to pass off faulty and limited information with an air of confidence. Still, browbeating days are over, and doctors are accustomed to descending from Olympian heights. Nevertheless, they may retain traces of an earlier dialectic, using special latinistic language that impresses and obfuscates.

I hope that someday legal contracts, insurance policies, and government documents will be intelligible enough to satisfy mere mortals seeking information and guidance lest they sign and agree to something in ignorance.

For purposes of self-instruction, seeking information should be preceded by foreknowledge that such information is trustworthy even if incomplete. This may require an act of faith, because authorities have been known to err widely and to insist loudly on their prerogatives.

The opposite or antithetical coping strategy is to be content, satisfied, and complacent. One patient said, "I don't need to know anything more about my illness. My doctor has told me everything, and I'm completely satisfied." When asked if she could report just what she understood and had been told, her information turned out to be very sketchy and uncertain, except that its effect was reassuring. Thus, she fended off a potential problem instead of coping with it. On the other hand, it is often unnecessary to imbue a patient with more information than can be used. This woman tended not to want specifics but to cope by passive acquiescence.

As a rule, the search for information and guidance is often spurred by a feeling that entrenched authority cannot be trusted absolutely. There are always crisp voices, flat declarations, and imperatives that intimidate the unwary, who are cowed into silent submission even when their life is on the line. We must insist that seeking information from reliable sources is a hard habit to acquire because it is far easier to get guidance and do what is expected without informed consent. When this occurs, we are not dealing with Coping Strategy 1 (CS 1) but with CS 8 or 12, to be explained in due time.

Coping strategy 2.
Share concern; find consolation

Mere information can be sought in books and maps as well as from other people. But finding information and exchanging experience is an important way of resonating with others. It is a *consoling* event to learn that one is not alone, that others understand a little, that consensus is established. Even the secret pleasure that many people get from spreading gossip can be traced to a desire to ostracize someone for having a fault or being caught at something we and others of similar high virtue would disparage.

Consolation means getting an ally to assuage our misery. The popularity of peer groups, consciousness-raising sessions, and many other organizations around a common theme of mutual misfortune is a testimony to the value of congeniality, which also may contribute to better definition and coping with a difficult, demoralizing misfortune.

But every coping strategy can be abused and faked. Sharing concern can be simulated when a person uses others merely as a sounding-board or as a conduit for discharging complaints. Nothing is learned; nothing is resolved; true shared appreciation of another person's plight is missing.

Psychiatrists are fully familiar with the patient who complains and complains without gaining any valid comprehension of the issues he complains about. When questioned, such people almost visibly draw a curtain across themselves, even diverting their eyes, as they wait for another opportunity for self-justification. Analogously, there are other patients who simply cannot share concern, and so consolation or comprehension comes with exceeding difficulty. They sit in granite silence, speaking but little and even then in catch-phrases and generalities. When they are able to complain or to present problems, they search not for valid information or even for consolation but only for ready-made formulas that would enable them to maintain distance, as before.

The antithetical strategy is used by people who value privacy, carefully nurturing a sense of independence even if erroneously, and resent intrusions. Ostensibly, they prefer to work things out alone.

The balanced opposition or dialectic in strategy between people who share concern and those who practice privacy illustrates how essential it is to avoid excessive reliance on one strategy or another. Taken to its extreme, any coping strategy precludes good coping. In all likelihood it is a defense against, rather than a coping with. Those who are usually called rigid, dogmatic, narrow-minded, and so forth are not just people who don't agree with our assumptions; they may be conspicuous examples of extreme reliance on only one or two strategies.

Not everything should be revealed or absolutely concealed

from others. Wisdom decides how much to disclose and share and when to remain aloof in closed conference with oneself. Either extreme can be abused, not used. The chronic confessor, the ear-bender, the self-righteous gadfly are familiar stereotypes who are just as objectionable as those who confuse stubborn silence with strength.

There is an existential concern about dissolution and loss of selfhood that underlies extreme versions of CS 2 and its antithesis. Dread of isolation can be as intimidating as fear that one yields or discloses too much when, out of loneliness, one person turns to another. Similarly, those who guard their privacy as if it were a precious gem may be concerned lest by sharing they are swallowed up by conventionality and ordinary values.

Obviously, neither extreme is disgraceful, only a bit risky. Together they comprise a significant strategy for getting along without losing personal status or melting into the crowd.

Coping strategy 3.
Laugh it off; change emotional tone

Laughter is an emotion, not by itself a strategy. Nevertheless, laughter can defuse a tense situation or, unfortunately, ignite one. It is possible to laugh for conflicting purposes: to heal, to hurt, to ridicule, to provide gentle relief.

For an emotion that seems lighthearted, laughing it off and changing the emotional tone of an urgent problem is very serious. It can be construed in different ways, but for the most part laughing it off permits a painful conflict or dysphoria to be carted away. As a rule, the dysphoria one dispenses with is anger and indignation, whether inside oneself or within another. I may laugh with embarrassment in talking about a situation I handled badly. I talk about it in order to share concern but also to get relief by unburdening myself and asking, in effect, "This wasn't so bad, was it?" I ask for tolerant amusement, not anger or indignation at my stupidity, nor ridicule and reproach.

Laughing-with and laughing-at are opposites, although the outward manifestation seems similar. Laughing at another is meant to ridicule; as a coping strategy, it disavows and distances oneself from a deplorable situation. Back in the thirties the Nazis were caricatured for a while, made fun of and joked about, until it got very serious and the plight of Jews became unbearable. Even today there are those addicted to ethnic jokes that presumably relieve tension or change the emotional tone of the antipathy felt by the joker. Like it or not, contempt for a special group, whether we sympathize with them or not, is a coping strategy that attempts to defuse and dissipate tension, animosity, and fear.

Freud hypothesized that jokes circumvent repression and allow the expression of forbidden topics. Consequently, many jokes deal with death, sexuality, perversion, excrement, and other matters deemed too disgusting, conflictual, or ghoulish for straight talk. But however appealing Freud's theory may be, it is a common finding that when a joke is explained, the result is not disgust, disdain, or dysphoria, but unmitigated boredom. Talking about a joke kills it. The element of surprise, with concomitant reversal of affect, is gone. People with much too much sorrow and sickness sometimes kid about their disability, without much participation by the listeners except to applaud their "courage" and marvel at their "good attitude."

The inner purpose of strategic laughter is to change one's attitude toward sickness, conflict, and pain. If nothing were forbidden or taboo and everything were out in the open, perhaps laughing, wit, and joking would then disappear or be repressed. The world might be a much meaner place than it already is.

There are, of course, some subjects and circumstances that make laughter or at least reduction in emotional tone seem scandalous or extremely hostile. In both cases retaliation would be invited. For example, one does not usually laugh at a funeral or in church. The emotional release, regardless of its benefit, might desecrate the occasion. But it is not because appropriate solemnity has been violated that people disapprove or are outraged. Laughing reverses or releases strong affect. Bereaved people would feel that their grief was being mocked or made light of; those in church might feel that their religious convictions were being scoffed at. I have personally never heard a joke about Auschwitz, but Jewish jokes that poke fun at so-called Jewish idiosyncrasies are a genre by themselves. The effectiveness of CS 3 depends on finding a tactful distance before the emotional tone can safely and discreetly be changed. When occasions are too heavy, solemn, and sacred, the light touch is as forbidden as the topics.

The antithesis of laughing it off is tedious, unplayful, lugubrious pedantry. Such heavy and humorless dehumanization makes a joke of itself. When a pedant picks over unimportant details, explains the obvious, uses up too much time, it is like a dog worrying a bone: much effort, little nourishment. Wit would dispense with the subject in a flash.

Coping strategy 4.
Forget it happened; put it out of your mind

Suppression is not only useful but at times vitally necessary. We cannot dwell incessantly on what cannot be coped with.

The key issue in CS 4, however, is not whether to forget something or deliberately dismiss it but how to decide which problems are worth dismissing until a later time, when another tactic could be used. It is obviously better to put aside a problem that nothing much can be done about than to fret futilely.

In general there are two kinds of conditions that cause distress but usually defy single-handed efforts to solve. In one we review an episode from the past in which we might have done things differently. This prompts shame and regret, and may even initiate a prolonged period of unresolved dysphoria. In the other typical condition, the problems are just too enormous, and we are too weak or in no position to influence events. For example, we may be highly aware of dangerous political trends, but aside from making points in discussion or contributing to committees that promise collective action, nothing can be done to advance our views.

Worry, without power to reverse the past or influence the future, poisons the will. In fact, worry itself can constitute a problem when it concentrates on minor issues or deals with matters too complicated and enormous. If important enough, such problems need other tactics than mere rumination. Consequently, effective coping demands that other strategies be found, so that intelligent alternatives that have a chance are not destroyed.

The purpose of strategic suppression is not to cultivate indifference but to facilitate selective attention to problems that can conceivably be influenced. Not many solutions to important problems are arrived at instantaneously, except in dreams. Inspiration is not as sudden as it seems; it is a feeling of exultation, not a strategy. A fresh viewpoint, after a period of deliberately using CS 4, may be more profitable than worry.

The strategy considered antithetical to suppression is hypervigilance. Worry means anxious, fruitless perseveration; hypervigilance means to be unusually alert for potential threat, for danger from unexpected sources. It has the same relation to suppression as having eyes everywhere to keeping eyes shut.

Although hypervigilance can be a respectable strategy for a short period, when carried to an extreme, it verges on panic. It is clearly impossible to heed every clue or to interpret every event as if it were a clue to a dangerous situation. For example, it is abundantly useful to look for unusual signs of toxicity when taking an unfamiliar medicine; side effects of drugs can be dangerous. But most of the time, despite occasional horror stories, medications have been adequately tested for toxicity, and side effects often are the price we pay for the therapeutic benefits. Pointless hypervigilance is blackmail to misfortune. Because it is largely unselective, it tends to numb sharpness and defeat true preparation for potential danger.

Nevertheless, to be alarmed is a natural response to nonspecific threats. Dread and worry often appear silently, not heralded by more than a desire to protect oneself against a number of antisurvival forces. The danger in *both* suppression and hypervigilance is to forget that we have options and choices, some of which are capable of controlling the risks and regrets that are rampant. Unless different strategies are tried, when a reasonable problem presents itself, the only outcome is lackluster apathy and surrender.

Coping strategy 5.
Keep busy; distract yourself

This strategy is so commonplace and its variations so hackneyed that the complexity of busyness and distraction as coping devices is easily overlooked. It is a natural consequence to CS 4, because forgetting is helped by doing something else that has little to do with the problem one wants to get away from.

What, for example, do cancer patients do after they are treated for their illness and return home? "There's no use worrying, so I had to get my mind off things and keep from feeling sorry for myself." "It was back to work, business as usual, just as if nothing had happened." "I decided to do something new. I volunteered at church; I never thought I'd ever do that!"

The important value in CS 5 is that concern is shifted to a nonproblem area. Because worry is vigilance spinning its wheels and boredom is suppression bringing every interest to a standstill, it is comforting and reassuring to find oneself able to maintain ordinary pursuits or even engage in new interests, business as usual, come what may.

However, keeping busy and being distracted is not the same as frittering away time doing nothing in particular. Puttering around is like digging a hole and filling it up again. Keeping busy in finding distraction or some other benefit when digging a hole is part of gardening, for example, or even ditchdigging. Keeping busy, not idling, requires a sense of purpose consistent with our dedication to benefit, even in our leisure.

What then is an appropriate antithetical strategy? Few people would admit to idling away time, except for very short periods and for very good reasons, so entrenched is the work ethic. Inactivity can, however, be a deliberate strategy, such as resting before the big game or closing the books before an examination. But these are studious pauses, posing as indulgences or even frivolity.

Aside from those few individuals who work hard at hedonism, there are other people who seemingly cultivate inactivity through pointless fantasies of someday, somehow, getting going, not unlike the barroom characters in *The Iceman Cometh* of O'Neill. Clearing the mind, waiting until one can look around, letting things settle are the tactical manifestations of being non-busy.

Beneath the problems of keeping busy, distracting oneself, and pausing before initiating a postponed action are problems of self-worth. Even a confirmed vagabond or tramp will at least talk about working or offer fabricated reasons for being nonproductive. The well-known distinction between a bum and dilettante is not merely their respective social standing but an attitude toward themselves. Many people wonder what work to do that will give them sufficient satisfaction as well as salary. But a more important existential question is "What am I capable of doing?" And within this question is another, "What am I afraid of doing and risking?"

These questions are urgent for those people who, for some reason, are abruptly fired, retired, or disabled, and no longer have any true responsibility. Their confusion concerns competence, morale, and personal worth. A child who has too many limits imposed and made to feel guilty at every turn toward developing autonomy has no room to grow. As a result, the busyness they develop is primarily noncontroversial and intentionally frivolous, although under the guise of following directions.

Coping strategy 6.
Confront the issue; act accordingly

This is the lodestone of coping strategies, because without being able to confront a problem and initiate appropriate action, coping is merely defensive retreat and avoidance. CS 6 is self-instruction's best ally. It summons and calls upon combinations of other strategies, thus showing versatility and flexibility at coping well. But it does not guarantee errorless behavior or faultless judgment—most people, most of the time, regard themselves as acting according to their "best judgment."

Those who characteristically confront problems also will consider consequences (CS10) and are neither impulsive nor dilatory. Nevertheless, to profess an ability or willingness to confront does not always mean straightforward and unequivocal behavior. There are always forces of self-deception pulling us away from self-realization. Honest self-appraisal, therefore, is a prerequisite; otherwise, those who pride themselves on being able to confront without hesitation may be afraid to acknowledge their limitations and the limitations of this proud strategy.

The term *confrontation* may need further clarification, since it is often confused with angry rebellion, taking a tough stand, challenging established authority, and so forth. Even in psychotherapy the word seems to suggest a demand for attention—"See here, you fool!" This is emphatically not my meaning. For me, confrontation is pointing someone toward a realization of a fact about himself or about the situation in which clarification is needed. Clarification should precede action, and what a good confrontation does is to make real the salient guidelines of a proposed action, even if it is to refrain and find another guideline.

Confrontation thrives on novelty; the tried and true method may only be the tedious and tired. Its antithesis is equivocation and procrastination. I do not suggest that confrontation followed by prompt action is always good or effective or that vacillation is always bad. He who hesitates may be lost but not more than he who plunges ahead heedlessly. In fact, those who procrastinate also may be concerned with short-term goals as well as long-range objectives.

Dreamers and idealists are indispensable counterbalances to the pragmatic confronters who briskly take action on problems as presented. While, from one viewpoint, dreamers and idealists look off at sea, waiting for ships that never come in, they also include creative spirits who may cope poorly with the near-at-hand while constructing a visionary grand design.

I doubt, however, whether truly creative spirits get very far by languishing amid clouds of speculation. They probably work just as hard (CS 5) in selecting, sorting, and revising hypotheses and arrangements of all kinds as do the more conspicuous copers.

The conflict between confrontation, productivity, and contemplation need not be resolved in one direction or another. Problem solving is not everything, and coping well is not and could not be the supreme value of human activity, because life is enriched by aesthetic, cultural, philosophical, and recreational pursuits that do not pay off by 'getting things done.' When one of the Ancients advised everything in moderation, it meant diversity in how one copes, even if the favorite strategy is confrontation.

Fear of fallibility is a key existential problem. Self-doubt turns a competent person into one who inflexibly hesitates, lest a mistake be made and blame be placed. That person is like a restricted child who worries about parental disapproval. The popular diagnosis, *midlife crisis*, is not confined to middle years nor is it a crisis. As a rule, it refers to self-made men who seemingly have been quite successful and have many reasons to be pleased with their progress—except that they are not. Suddenly they become unsure of what they want and what to do next. Instead of confronting issues and acting accordingly, they vacillate; customary values shuffle about aimlessly and even dissolve. Wealth, position, respect, family ties, love, all dwindle. Such people also require other coping strategies besides that of confrontation.

Coping strategy 7.
Redefine; take a more sanguine view

In order to optimize a plight and reduce distress, it is often useful to redefine and rise above a difficult problem. Unless a person rises above discouragement and potential failure, he may quickly sink below and be engulfed by further difficulties.

At issue in the strategy of redefinition is that peculiarly indefinable trait called *heart*. Psychology makes much of those who are disheartened but tends to overlook how one takes heart and is heartened by.

Heart means courage, but CS 7 means more than having fortitude or being optimistic. These are hardly strategies but dispositions and moods—they may result from taking heart or being encouraged. In general, to redefine means to make a virtue out of necessity, turn coercion into a choice, transform a deficit into a gain, and make unpleasantness tolerable. The joke about the man who fell downstairs and then said he was going down anyway is an example of redefining a plight in acceptable terms. The half-empty, half-full bottle is equally familiar. CS 7 is a way of turning an unhappy situation into one that can be coped with because the distress is reduced.

One can redefine and rise above in many ways. Tact, diplomacy, courtesy, euphemism are all examples of looking at a plight and softening its impact. Frequently, arguments can be defused by redefining the situation in such a way that permits the combatants to save face without giving up their viewpoints. "There has been an unfortunate misunderstanding here. I am sure that whatever problems exist can be settled." "No, we are not firing you, but we believe that another person would work better within our organization at this particular time."

Redefinition takes a more sanguine view by other than verbal means; humor also is effective. This is not reversal of affect, as in CS 3, but a more relaxed attitude that gently accepts misunderstanding and cools tempers.

The best redefinitions are those that seem very natural. A soft answer turneth away wrath, and a soft sell works best when the customer believes the article is just what he needs. Every psychotherapist of quality knows this strategy. Such therapists can be both sanguine and straightforward, presenting a thought gently but firmly. Pollyanna, the eternal optimist, never admits a problem, and is not, therefore, a strategist. Her descendants, the very positive thinkers so admired a generation ago, visualize only very positive outcomes, never the possibility of failure. CS 7 does not deceive anyone but tends to make coping more feasible, and more likely. It can be cultivated, and when sufficiently practiced, the adept strategist will develop more positive expectations. If he or she is a psychotherapist or anyone who deals with people in a considerate fashion, empathy itself may be encouraged.

A cancer patient refused treatment, saying that he had never been sick before and didn't plan on being sick now. He had heard that cancer treatment made people sick, so it was not for him.

His logic was sound, but his definition of sickness needed redefinition along with a more sanguine view. He did not dwell on having cancer; he wanted only to stay well and had no intention of damaging his health by treatment. The consultant used CS 7 in persuading the patient to *choose* treatment in order to ensure continued good health and not allow the cancer to undermine his well-being. In other words, as the patient viewed the problem, avoidance was preferred, but the problem would not go away. As the consultant worked it out, the patient was encouraged to use CS 6 along with CS 7.

The most favorable version of CS 7 is one that "optionizes" or "optimizes" a problem, without compromising truth or promulgating an illusion. Thus, it fosters firmer morale.

There are two ways in which redefinition and taking a more sanguine view find their opposites. One common strategy is avoidance; the other is deliberately to adopt a pessimistic attitude. The latter sometimes is called "bitter truth," "worst possible scenario," or "straight-from-the-shoulder." Curiously, these two antitheses of redefinition are in themselves polar opposites! Avoidance has hardly anything to recommend it, except that it might minimize needless fretting. Pessimizing, however, could force someone to prepare for a bleak future, since optimism, comfortable or not, also needs resources to work well.

Sad to say, there are many people who work hard at earning the merits of defeat and find success to be an uneasy victory. Like some perverse alchemist, they turn gold into lead. They may offer much to others but insist that nothing be asked of them because they feel unable to fulfill expectations. Their self-esteem is precarious, and pessimism seems to be a natural consequence of making any effort. To find life smooth sailing is disturbing. In their attitude of surrender, the outlook is based on vigilant preparation for a shipwreck.

Coping strategy 8.
Resign yourself; make the best of what can't be changed

Although life is not quite as bleak as it is for those preparing for a shipwreck, those who use CS 8 seek resignation to a plight or problem, not redefinition (CS 7).

Submission to defeat is a dismal consequence, not a strategy. It is not the same as strategic resignation and making the best of what can't be changed. CS 8 is a choice that is intended to acknowledge forces beyond control. Resignation has a long, honorable history in many fields. It is linked to the tradition of stoicism and mysticism. Acquiescence to the mystery of the world need not be an attitude of passive surrender or capitulation. The truly resigned will concede that there are immutable, incomprehensible forces as well as eternal questions for which no answer is likely to be found. This can be a somewhat exalting experience.

Ordinary people are, as a rule, neither stoics nor mystics, nor, for that matter, do they assiduously seek rational information. Cancer patients commonly say, "There's nothing more for me to do but wait and see." To wait and see can mean resignation, but it is also a strategy that counsels postponement, not unlike CS 4.

The antithesis of resignation and making the best of a situation often amounts to the same thing, as in the case of a man who one day decided that he had had enough tests, operations, and transfusions for too little lasting benefit. He wanted no more, and said so. While he was subdued, he was by no means ready to capitulate. His choice was resignation (CS 8) but also one of dispassionate *rebellion*. Together, these two antithetical strategies amounted to a decision not to comply with what was expected of him.

Behavior of this sort shows how difficult it is to select one and only one strategy out of many, without fully understanding the context in which an individual asserts his or her right to choose. Even resignation, as much as rebellion, declares an option, "I must do this in order to be myself, keep self-respect, knowing that I can endure even if things cannot be changed."

Coping strategy 9.
Do something, anything, perhaps exceeding good judgment

In the example cited above, the patient issued an existential ultimatum: No more treatment; I must be myself regardless of what my doctors think.

Doing something, anything, even in excess of the norm, and perhaps going beyond the prudent judgment of most people, hardly seems like a strategy worth opting for. Yet this is what many decide. "What do I have to lose?" "I can't stand this uncertainty!" While it may be bravado, or more often, despair, CS 9 means, "What else can I lose beyond what is already gone?" or "Unless I do something, I shall surely be lost!"

Naturally, few people undertake an action knowing that it is foolhardy or impulsive. These are afterthoughts. Most people believe that their behavior is within rational bounds of good judgment, even if similar conduct has led to trouble in the past. A gambler, accustomed to losing, still seeks the elusive "big score." Exhibitionists, one must presume, are driven to expose themselves in busy places and, at least consciously, hope not to be caught.

The most common example of CS 9 is the use and abuse of alcohol. It is significant that many heavy drinkers are almost arrogant in declaring their ability to hold and control the amount they consume, thus indicating a choice or pseudochoice. With this declaration they imply that the amount is within normal limits. Drinking is thus a coping strategy, designed to help people be sociable, relaxed, calm, all traits approved by the community's customs.

Good reasons are seldom hard to find; correct reasons are more difficult. Consequently, alcohol abusers may never find it convenient to abstain, even if they drink to excess in everyone's eyes except their own. Under the influence, alcohol abusers try to feel the way they think ordinary people are expected to feel or be without excessive drinking or self-destructive behavior.

To do something, anything, even at the risk of exceeding good judgment is a strategy intended to resolve problems without delay; normalcy is taken by storm or at least simulated. CS 9, therefore, is intended to concoct normality, often enough through concoctions of one kind or another—e.g., alcohol, drugs, tobacco, fighting, fornication—clearly in excess.

Abstinence, the antithesis of CS 9, also can be carried to excessive extremes. It refers to the use and abuse of normalcy and morality, as if the choice of disciplined behavior means to equate normal behavior with high morality. Consequently, abstemious conduct is often self-righteous, as if the individual sets the standard for the community.

Like many other paired opposite strategies, excessive action and disciplined abstinence have much in common. Puritanical joy in virtue has its own flush of excitement, fully as intoxicating as a man who feels completely in control after a few drinks but much wittier, thoughtful, amorous, articulate than if he had had nothing. The common theme shared by abstinence and abuse is an attempt to contain and control tendencies to life-threatening behavior. Their common aim is to make life seem better than it is.

I cannot agree with Camus that suicide is a principal philosophic problem. However, life-threatening and dangerous behavior is often an intriguing dark shadow behind many efforts to cope with problems. A young college student was accustomed to putting himself to the test of courage by deliberately taking chances. He would dive into shallow water, ski over unknown trails, drive his car fast, and one night, while feeling particularly uneasy and inadequate, he jumped from a fifth-floor window. Through no fault of his, he struck an awning, breaking the fall, and survived. He reported that for one brief moment, just before he began to fall, he had the ecstatic sensation of being completely free and unencumbered by the world and his worries. In an existential sense, he could fly—until, of course, gravity took over.

Coping strategy 10.
Review alternatives; examine consequences

That poets seem to die so often by their own decree and design is a perplexing and tragic mystery that I do not pretend to understand. Perhaps they do not kill themselves more frequently than do professors, teachers, or dentists. Perhaps it seems that way because poets epitomize sensitivity and spontaneity, as well as having high verbal skills. Suicide, therefore, may represent both dread of losing talent and vanishing sensitivity. At bottom, this is fear of insanity, an existential state with which poets may be conspicuously familiar.

Review of alternatives in a proposed action is anything but spontaneous and enthusiastic behavior. Action is postponed until consequences can be examined and evaluated. It seems so reasonable and rational that hardly anyone would object. But therein are the difficulties.

If a person delays making a decision too long, the strategy may backfire and end in vacillation. If review of alternatives is too brief, the ensuing action might be considered rash and reckless, especially if things go wrong. How long is long enough? In an action-oriented society, mulling over various options is pretty dull and may even be an excuse for not acting at all. For example, a young man who endlessly reviews the qualities he wants in a wife is probably not very eager to be married in the first place. The essential ingredient of caring for someone enough to overlook her shortcomings is missing.

CS 10 need not be a stodgy search for safe alternatives. It does mean thinking things through, and this can be accomplished swiftly or deliberately, depending on the problem and its consequences. There is a wide difference between saving a child from drowning and preparing a research protocol. The urgency and complexity of a situation will call for different kinds of review.

The opposite strategy is to act out of habit, without much forethought for consequences. When earlier strategies have worked well enough with similar problems, why change? When a doctor calls upon his "clinical experience," he intends to remain loyal to beliefs, methods, and medication that have served him and his patients well. Not every problem is so noteworthy or urgent that it deserves radical alteration in management or even serious, prolonged reflection. Innovation for its own sake or to preen oneself on being "modern" is usually a superfluous posture, teaching us very little about either the problem or effective coping methods.

CS 10 means rational reflection, timed and executed according to the urgency of the problem. Its opposite is not irrationality or confusion but an equally concise pattern of following well-trod paths. If there is an underlying existential concern shared by CS 10 and its antithesis, it is one that asks: Where are we going?

What is worth doing? How shall we find out? There are several paths I could follow, but where do they lead?

Our contemporary cry for "self-identity" is simply an updated version of a much older problem of salvation. What should I care about and dare to act upon? This is a more important question than to be or not to be.

A child will ask, "What will I be when I grow up?" A young adult will wonder what the future holds. A more settled, middle-aged person may fret, "Is this what I am? Could anything have been different?" A much older person's question is "What has been worth doing? How have I measured out my life?" Review of alternatives can be brief and trivial or so extensive as to encompass the purpose of having lived. We puzzle over our freedom and autonomy without wholly ignoring the possibility that we are simply an ingenious biological phenomenon with a peculiar sense of its own existence.

Coping strategy 11.
Get away from it all; find an escape, somehow

What if . . .
Regardless of how well one copes and contends with problems, most efforts to instruct oneself come down to asking what if something else had happened, some other path had been followed, different events had determined another course. "What if" is an inevitable question that is of necessity incomplete and unanswerable.

Who can honestly claim never to have thought about the "paths not taken"? Who can claim never to have wanted simply to get away from a nagging, seemingly insoluble problem? A middle-aged housewife, mother of three children, had recently been diagnosed as having metastatic cancer. She was in considerable pain and feared the inevitable outcome. Although married to a devoted husband, she did recall attending summer school many years before and spending a few afternoons with a young Mexican exchange student. Her shyness and conservatism kept her from going beyond friendly chats, but now she wondered, "What if I had been able to have an affair with him?" If she only had a week or two, could she have known what a different life was like?

Basically, she would not have changed the way her life turned out, but obviously she retained the fantasy of getting away from her conventional life and finding some of the passionate fulfillment that her husband and children did not provide.

Ishmael immortalizes the man who copes with the damp, drizzly November in his soul by getting away, finding escape, somehow, from something unnamed. His route was hardly a vacation, but his strategy was CS 11. Others have their own hiding places, secret grottos, where they escape, replenish their spirit, and find change of heart, until the turmoil of being alive abates.

The antithesis is to stay put, see things through, stick it out, hang on, and in general endure tenaciously. But retreat does not necessarily include surrender to an insoluble problem. Certain reprieves are almost medicinal. What matters is to escape from imprisoning and exhausting circumstances. However, not every escape gets away from the pursuit of what was left behind. There are fugitives always and everywhere, vainly trying to get away from no one except themselves. Their strategy is mistaken, and the antithesis, coupled with better self-instruction, might be more successful.

Coping strategy 12.
Conform, comply; do what is expected or advised

Because most people regularly do it, and everyone does it much of the time, this strategy carries its own justification. It is comfortable, and more passive than the previous strategies. While conformity has a superficial resemblance to resignation (CS 8), they are much different in that resignation may be rueful acquiescence to what can't be changed, while compliance seems altogether natural and hardly a strategy. A young man who goes into a thriving family business may not be in any doubt at all; he does what is expected and advised and will probably do the same thing in most important life decisions. When we consult a broker, he tells us how to invest, just as a doctor advises about what ails us and what to do about it. Generally, we comply, because compliance is expected of us, quite apart from whether the information we seek (CS 1) or the concern we share (CS 2) is sufficient.

CS 12 applies mostly in fields that we know little about and rely on expert opinions and opinionated experts. To rely on rules and conventional pathways is to ensure getting along, not getting away, because only a few people are able to act wholly independently without the sanction of acceptance and approval. If the restrictions set by conformity and compliance are not overly rigid and confining, we are not offended or compromised. It does not mean intimidation, obedience, or capitulation. Nevertheless, unless one watches out, doing what is expected might become "Take it or leave it; comply, don't complain!"

The opposite of conformity and compliance is certainly not criminality. I cannot hazard a surmise about what goes on in the mind of a total criminal, whether murderer or swindler. But sin is not very original, and criminal offenses are as stereotyped as the most straightforward behavior of the most law-abiding citizen. I suspect that chronic law-breakers may be ultraconformists at heart, true to their own values and responding with strategies that are advocated or accepted by the group with which they feel affiliated.

The difference between sin, vice, and crime may be psychologically very slight or very broad, depending on the perpetrator and those who make the distinction. Conformity and compliance are strategies, because even if we rebel against rules and expectations, we specifically disavow certain rules, and are not totally negativistic. When we are sick and confined to a hospital, we are exempted from some rules but expected to conform to the sick role. A good patient complies, does not ask many questions, goes along with inconvenience, and is expected to get well, pay the bill, and be very appreciative. Compliance will assure reasonable care, security, and enough respect to tolerate the indignities of hospitalization. But too much acquiescence is not wise, neither is it respected. Those who are poor, ignorant, inept, and disabled gain very little from their disadvantage in our society. They submit because they have so little power to retaliate, rebel, or cause trouble.

The true opposite of CS 12 is conspicuous deviation from the norm or from adherence to rules, which is not, as I have already noted, identical with chronic criminality. A noisy maverick violates expectations, but a fanatic who seemingly deviates from the norm may only exaggerate conventional morality. To evangelize is to urge an ultraorthodoxy or return to rudimentary values. Acquiescence and assertion contribute to a delicate formula for healthy autonomy. One need not be a George Babbitt when complying with social expectations, nor a George Orwell when defying the establishment. The wise counsel is to pick the place to take a stand and choose the cause that can be defended.

Norms and expectations, rules and regulations, customs and conventions are not necessarily vicious or antisurvival. Society, at least in broad perspective, sets standards and limits that are designed to protect us from each other. Compliance, under many circumstances, is a choice that is not only prudent but may even require more courage than simple deviant behavior.

The real question is how far and how long we should comply and conform, do what is expected, or depend on advice before we declare we have had enough of whatever it is. Tell me not what is good for me unless you first say what is good for you.

Coping strategy 13.
Blame or shame someone, something

Blaming or shaming someone or something for a problem or predicament goes on practically all the time. Yet few people will admit this as a favorite strategy, although its intention is to exonerate them from responsibility.

Perhaps the reader has already noticed that in my arrangement of common coping strategies I have listed them so that each strategy deals with leftover elements of the strategy preceding it. Consequently, blaming or shaming someone assigns fault for a misfortune somewhere outside, probably because we have a sense of having failed to meet inner expectations or standards.

Gossip could not be as enjoyable as it is without exculpating those who gossip from a similar offense, whatever it is. However, when CS 13 gets out of control, the result may be paranoia or melancholia, maybe both. I am bad, but you are worse, You abuse me, but I deserve no better.

Often, the person who is a chronic loser will blame and seek to shame others for failure and misfortunes. How often do we hear people blaming parents, spouses, jobs, or minorities for their inadequacies or renunciation of responsibility?

Although certain depressed patients show a kind of arrogance and egotism about just who is the most evil and unworthy, it is a mistake to think of blame and shame as pathological. The pseudoarrogance of a melancholic or paranoid patient comes, I think, from his or her social conformity to group values and expectations. There is a self-righteousness that shines through efforts to deplore.

Consequently, the opposite strategy of CS 13 is refusal to retaliate, point the finger, or seek to impose punishment. I can find no other designation but the very loaded term *forgiveness*. As a rule, to forgive is considered a high virtue or a sign of stupidity. We can scarcely believe it when someone says, "I decided to forgive and forget." How is it possible to transmute hostility into something akin to neutrality, and then forget it all? In most cases, I notice, forgiveness is a strategy in which one puts retaliation aside because the issue is not worth the effort or risk of further alienation. Moreover, suppressing anger may have some recompense in not creating a permanent grievance or enmity.

The concern behind blame or shame is not altogether a wish for forgiveness or exculpation. It is fear of indifference. We want others to notice and care for us through their approval and acceptance. Similar intentions are also behind jealousy, envy, and self-pity. I am jealous of the man she loves instead of me. I envy those who have had it better. I pity myself for not being better loved, taken care of, or endowed with superior talents. Socialization and civility, of course, teach us to forswear jealousy, envy, and self-pity. But we retain traces, often very strong traces, of resentment when someone seemingly has it better, and we, by comparison, are treated with indifference and neutrality.

We talk on about "fairness," when there is little evidence of even apportionment and allotment of love, talent, or money. The existential crime that worries us is that offenders go unpunished, witnesses look the other way, and that we are basically as indifferent as anyone else who does not want to get involved.

Much has been written about a nebulous concept called *existential guilt*. Are we at fault for being born? I find no place for existential guilt within the concept of responsibility. Instead, I think it belongs to how we ordinarily deal with unjustifiable human suffering. We dread indifference and neutrality in others but are largely apathetic to their plight. How much pain is enough before we feel guilty for not caring enough? When do we deserve forgiveness?

Coping strategy 14.
Give vent; feel emotional release

When tension mounts or protests go unvoiced and unheeded, sometimes there is no other non-tantrum tactic but to let go. This may consist of a good cry, brief ranting and raving, sullen withdrawal, or any other modality in which giving vent to strong emotion under more or less controlled circumstances is strategic.

While not every problem is readily solved, to put it very mildly, there are many ways to find emotional decompression. Substance intake or emotional catharsis will lower the level of tension. To ventilate a grievance is more specific, because giving vent by itself is simply to discharge feeling.

Giving vent is either an act of catharsis or a strategy. If the latter, there is an implied element of control. As a rule, this needs an accepting environment in which no permanent rift or damage is incurred. For example, booing and hissing are part of the spectacle at sporting events. But attacking the referee is unacceptable. The idea behind an accepting environment is that an outburst will be condoned, even encouraged, provided that it is not destructive. In short, giving vent is really controlled deflation of distress.

The primary difference between catharsis and control depends on regulated discharge of strong feeling. Most of the regulation comes from awareness of social sanction or implied limits. There is a psychiatric theory that anger and grief need to be fully expressed, lest some dire disease result. However, no psychiatrist to my knowledge has encouraged patients to voice or act out their rage and grief except under specified controlling conditions, such as an office or at home, where forgiveness is supposed to be readily obtainable. There is a sanction that controls giving vent.

A man was severely criticized for flying into a rage at his wife, who was in the hospital dying of cancer. The staff considered him not only callous but cruel. Nevertheless, he told me later that at night when everyone in the family was asleep, he would go into the garage and weep bitter tears of protest, helplessness, and suffering. He could not control anger at his wife, however, because the sight of her suffering generated too much frustration. Rage at his wife created only more frustration, no relief, whereas his bouts of crying at night at least permitted him to sleep. Had he *blamed* his wife for being ill and dying, this would have been CS 13.

The opposite strategy also requires a certain positioning between catharsis, social sanction, and control, except that the appropriate emotion is strongly inhibited but not dismissed. This is a key difference from CS 4.

CS 14 raises a basic existential question of how much disclosure is permissible. Even the angry husband who seemed and probably was cruel to his wife contained himself enough to be alone at night before weeping so profusely. We talk much about social support and sharing concerns, but are we endangered by revealing highly personal feelings without first filtering them through customs and conventions?

Were we wholly candid and truthful at all times, a great many people would be unnecessarily alienated, and not much would be accomplished. Protest is certainly permissible, and maybe it is healthful, but only with a stipulation that, having given vent, we can be restored to regulated society again.

Coping strategy 15.
Deny as much as possible

I have deliberately left denial for the end of my list. Negation *almost* completes the circle of strategies that began with seeking information and sharing concern, and now terminates with fulsome denial.

Ordinary parlance systematically reveals and conceals, mixing forthright declarations with irrelevances, euphemisms, and downright fabrication. Just as we sometimes restrain conduct in the interest of civilized behavior, human interaction needs many kinds of accommodation, including liberal use of negation, distortion, and denial.

Denying as much as possible is a strategy that specifically disavows information by using negative terms. Obvious facts are culled, unfavorable implications are concealed, and unacceptable consequences are ignored. The purpose of blanket denial is to preserve a situation as it is, or would be, unchanged, but perhaps even better.

Denying as much as possible means to affirm or declare as little as possible, since no speech is entirely free of its negations. "As much as possible" is intended to keep everything in order as long as possible. The staunch denier will, understandably, present himself in somewhat idealized and unnatural terms. "No, I'm not sick. In fact, I'm rarely sick at all." "No, I have never even looked at another woman besides my good wife." "I don't know what the fuss is all about, or why the family even wanted to know if I'm okay!"

Ignorance and lack of information are not the same as denial, but failure to seek information supports denying. Consequently, denying is largely a social strategy that would preserve things as they were or might be. Unfortunately, professionals often speak about the "mechanism of denial" as if it were a kind of switch that could be turned off and on. As a social strategy, denying depends on what is denied, and when, how, and to whom the denial is expressed. One might be quite candid with an old friend but cautious and reserved to the point of denying as much as possible with a stranger, such as a doctor or nurse. Or it could be the other way round when a person wants to preserve a relationship with an old friend but has no stake in fabricating with a professional.

Denying as *much* as possible closes off the world of uncertainty and fragility, of fickleness and distress. As a result, it is difficult to develop self-instruction or good coping strategies. Denial does have a place in the way we modulate distress or control stimuli that might hurt. Selective attention to certain facts and avoidance of others may even point to new options, but to do so, attention, not iron-clad denial, is required. After all, we must acknowledge that a problem or dilemma exists before it can be coped with. A healthy autonomy will starve on a diet of strict denial, but excessive candor may be equally unpalatable, especially if it filters out compassion.

I do not strongly object to denial as such but to the company it keeps: avoidance, escapism, self-deception, and so on. Denying, even as much as possible, does have a strategic and existential value, albeit quite temporary. We may not think very highly of ourselves, with our shabby and selfish motives, but we cannot afford to think less of ourselves and let others know about it indiscriminately. Self-deception is a common vice; innocent deception of others could almost be a virtue. It might be part of self-instruction. Since we are on guard much of the time, self-doubt can be answered by any affirmation that gives us the benefit of the doubt. Consequently, those who use denying as much as possible for inordinately protracted periods are probably deeply concerned about their self-worth and endangerment.

This list is both too long and too short. But the strategy of coping is seldom simple, unambiguous, and plain. Even major strategies borrow and attach themselves to others and need dissection to be better understood. Coping with hunger, for example, involves much more than foraging for food. There are social, ethical, economic, aesthetic, and physical considerations, as well as certain skills related to cooking, paying for, and sharing different kinds of food. And this is a very fundamental problem, far easier to deal with than more complex issues.

Those who cope well tend to use a wider range of strategies, while specializing in the strategies they know most about. Self-instruction depends on discovering new resources and perfecting what has worked reasonably well in the past. How we cope with any problem, what action we take, will inevitably change the nature of that problem, recasting it in copable or at least familiar terms.

CHAPTER 4

BETWEEN VULNERABILITY AND MORALE

The ancient Stoics would not need me to explain that there is much virtue in necessity and considerable vice in freedom. Habit, duty, and obligation can spare us much indecision and anguish, while freedom without discipline is often a source of mischief.

Freedom in the sense of being able to choose between alternatives, or even in the sense of feeling free, is a perplexing phenomenon. At times it is an illusion; but elsewhere it is one of our most precious commodities. It is an essential ingredient for cultivating and strengthening coping strategies. Because there is little genuine freedom to spare, we need to use it well.

I have already emphasized that with so much anxiety about survival, ambivalence in our deepest relationships, and ambiguity in what we understand and do, hardly anyone can be expected to cope superlatively at all times. Many human problems have no discernible solutions. Our morale and self-esteem are exposed to a variety of erosions and explosions, and distress is almost a natural state of being.

Nevertheless, between extreme vulnerability and high morale, most of us manage to get by, using a mixture of habit and improvisation. We develop a set of useful strategies that works well enough to keep death and self-destruction at a safe distance.

Coping well enough depends on having adequate resources that both supply basic needs and permit personal development. Psychosocial adaptation is based on the reciprocal interaction between effective coping strategies and susceptible vulnerability. If coping goes well, morale is lifted; if not, then vulnerability imposes and exposes us to manifold forces of evil.

The epitome of bad coping, high vulnerability, and low morale is suicide. While numerous people daily perpetrate self-destructive acts, their reasons are barely plausible and not very convincing. I do not have a comprehensive theory of what prompts people to attempt or commit suicide, but then I cannot collect a persuasive set of arguments for staying alive. At many moments life and its incessant troubles seem like a losing cause. The effort makes very little sense. But whether the argument is to live or die, rationality lets us down. Although being alive has fluctuating value or purpose in the emotional marketplace, most people, regardless of their personal dismay, manage to retain a trace of competence, control, and composure.

PRECEPTS FOR GOOD COPING

What do good copers do that bad or mediocre copers do not? Different problems call for different sets of primary strategies, yet good copers manage to deal with problems in similar ways that are more effective than those of bad copers.

Because these strategies can be learned, I present the more successful tactics in a somewhat pedagogical fashion. It is not meant to be dictatorial; these are precepts to be used and modified, as needed.

(1) Confront problems as directly as possible. Revisions and corrections will be necessary because intermediate issues need coping with first, step by step, before larger issues can be tackled.

(2) Look for reliable information and, when needed, find and use trustworthy support. It is also important to know that not all support is helpful and may even be detrimental. You may have to go it alone.

(3) Keep communication reasonably open with significant key others, but remember that *you* are the key support, so deserve your trust.

(4) Learn to know the difference between guidance and advice. When advice is to ignore your preferences, be cautious about following that advice. People may push you to do what *they* want.

(5) There is nothing holy or certain about what you want, and while choice is your option, compliance is not always misleading.

(6) Even professional help can be questioned. Make sure of its quality, regardless of the job to be done. Most people are, understandably, mainly altruistic on their own behalf. Ask who is being helped to what.

(7) If possible, choose an active strategy, but carefully. Do not depend on vacuous reassurance that all will be well, and that nothing further need be done except to wait patiently. Nevertheless, just as relaxation stores up energy and revives the tired spirit, quiet reflection may be more productive than feverish, poorly thought through action.

(8) Besides the capacity to cope, one often needs the courage to cope. After all, even with the best intention, information, preparation, and resourcefulness, you can be wrong. You can falter and be misled. Good copers do not always succeed.

(9) Good coping is seldom effective when one is agitated, alarmed, angry, or in the throes of an extreme emotion. Composure and compassion are bound to be beneficial, except, of course, in certain emergencies.

(10) Distress means that a problem is still active and

uncoped with. Learn to tolerate distress while coping with it.

VULNERABILITY AND WHAT IT MEANS

Insofar as we fall short of understanding what anything important means, we are vulnerable, though perhaps not distressed. Nevertheless, in the search for meaning, the meaning of vulnerability is a critical task.

It is a curious yet recurrent observation that the truly significant concepts we deal with are difficult to define, as if we are too immersed in the actions and connotations they evoke. Nevertheless, most of us know by instinct, intuition, or some other native faculty what an idea that evokes strong emotion feels like. Therefore, we are led to behave in certain ways that show a deeper sense of meaning than carefully chosen words and abstractions can convey. Vulnerability is such a concept.

First, I find it useful to divide any meaning into three parts: *objective, organic*, and *surplus*. *Objective meaning* is a categorical feature belonging to a public reality. Such meanings appear in dictionaries and are used intelligibly in sentences, permitting people to communicate reasonably well. *Organic meaning* is a guide for action or an operation, suggesting a certain type of behavior. It refers primarily to what is done or could be performed. *Surplus meaning* refers to the private significance of an object, directly experienced by an individual but difficult to share.

Because this description of meaning has an *external reference point*, it is somewhat easier to understand than more personal or existential meanings. For example, a pocket watch may be defined as an instrument that divides the day and night into equal intervals. This is true for all timepieces and thus is its *objective* meaning.

If a watch, particularly this watch, is defined as a portable device that permits me to "tell time" and be prompt for appointments, I am speaking of its *organic* meaning.

When I speak of this watch only, I may describe it as the pocket watch my father gave me on his deathbed, telling me to take good care of it, since it was very expensive. This is the *surplus* meaning that matters only to me. It is one of a kind. It retains the same surplus meaning, apart from its time-telling function or objective resemblance to other timepieces, whether it works or not.

In the world of private experience the dictionary lets us down. Definitions of beauty, sorrow, pity, and so on are pretty meager. The meaning of vulnerability, according to Webster, is the state or quality of being vulnerable. Vulnerable means "capable of being wounded" or "liable to attack or injury." Both of these have an *external* reference, just as their synonyms—*defenseless; exposed*—imply an external attack.

The objective meaning of vulnerability is, therefore, negligible. Its force comes from organic and surplus meaning, although defenseless against attack does refer to an outside injury. The organic activity related to vulnerability is a disposition to act or behave in a way that reflects an inner distress. The surplus meaning of vulnerability is at the core of the experience. Most such experiences are conveyed with difficulty, but to save us from a total absorption with our own inner sentiments, language combines internal and external reference points. Words are almost always symbols or signs that require inferences, even about the most concrete object or thing. The more unique or idiosyncratic our language becomes, the more it is trying to express the totally subjective. One of the genuine obstacles to psychoanalytic research, for example, is that psychoanalysis lacks a common observational language for internal experiences. What patients say are hypotheses and interpretations of private emotions and external psychosocial situations.

Communication depends on a consensus between people with respect to the organic meaning of events. It is a shared experience. Then, after the event is sufficiently talked about, we arrive at a paraphrase of what we already know, and this becomes the objective meaning that appears in dictionary definitions and sounds so redundant.

My grief over the death of someone I love is highly private and cannot be shared. It is one of a kind. What friends observe is behavior that, to them, is a distress signal. The organic meaning of my grief is my behavior, although the surplus meaning of what is called my grief is a feeling conveyed only by a series of approximations and synonyms: loss, emptiness, sadness, and so forth. The objective meaning of grief is a further inference, drawn from other people whose behavior reflects an inner dysphoria. That some observers consider *grief* to be the synonym for sorrow, sense of loss, bereavement, or mourning is, to be logical and psychological about it, their privilege of combining a variety of behavior related to death, desertion, damage.

With these ground rules for deciding what a painful emotion is and leads to, vulnerability has two important meanings: (a) a sense of immediate suffering (surplus meaning), and (b) a tendency to behave and act in certain ways that either express the feeling of suffering or designate attempts to get rid of it. The first meaning is called *dysphoria*; the second, *disposition*.

Strong emotion in itself is not necessarily a sign of distress and vulnerability. Love can be quite pleasant at times, and the aesthetic experience associated with art and fine music often is exalting. Furthermore, one can be very sensitive to distress and still cope well. In fact, anyone who claims never to feel vulnerable is no more to be believed than if he said he had never felt a strong emotion. Vulnerability, in my sense, is largely confined to the more distressing emotions that are usually strong enough to be noticed and responded to.

A common example of dysphoria is *embarrassment*, an emotion more common than grief, less common than anger, more individualistic than either. Embarrassment is a transitory suffering in the presence of others that is usually followed by a disposition to move away and retreat to a less threatening but more familiar situation. Other common dysphorias include such feelings as jealousy, boredom, disgust, astonishment, complacency, and so on, none of which are as strong and undifferentiated as emotional extremes (rage, panic, despondency).

There is, of course, a universe of major, minor, and moderate vulnerabilities. A thousand little pigments color our emotional life, and they inevitably contribute their portion to how we act, are acted upon, and cope. Generally, however, the more dysphoric the emotion, the less effective is our disposition to cope with whatever problem evoked a response. Indeed, this law of inverse relationship between coping and vulnerability allows us to measure effectiveness by means of scales that measure intensity and type of distress.

Textbooks and clinical manuals struggle with the task of differentiating between major dysphorias, but psychotherapists of quality seek to understand varying hues of mood and do distinguish between different dysphorias such as embarrassment, sarcasm, bitterness, and so on. Nevertheless, in everyday practice, many therapists and clinicians oversimplify emotional states and try to reach an objective meaning by ignoring qualitative differences between feelings. A good example is *depression*.

A patient may have private feelings of dejection, discouragement, loss of energy, or apathy, he may feel only a sense of ennui, or he may back away from any challenge, pleading belief in absolute failure. The range of dysphoria in what is called depression covers much of the emotional field. Clinicians may notice that a patient also sleeps poorly, eats hardly at all, broods by himself, and is sexually uninterested. He may ply himself with sundry medications or even consider self-destruction.

Details and individuated differences in dysphorias and dispositions are pushed aside in order to "objectify" a class of people into a class of events, collectively called depression. Surplus meaning is ignored, and organic meaning of behavior is shoved into a slot of pseudo-objective meaning. I submit that this is an upside-down way to understand very private dysphoria. It seems to me that vulnerability, consisting of both dysphoria and disposition, covers a variety of existential plights, in which one's reality as a person is threatened with special kinds of demoralization. In the following section I shall illustrate how we can start with surplus meaning, then include the organic meaning of various dispositions, and finally attempt an overall characterization of the plight without ignoring the uniqueness of the situation for an individual.

FOUR EXISTENTIAL PLIGHTS

Vulnerability is predicated on helplessness and hopelessness, even to the point that insofar as a person feels that he lacks hope and feels demoralized, that point determines whether he is confronted with a major, moderate, or minor vulnerability.

Poets and patients know all too well how difficult it is to convey an inner emotion adequately and to translate their sense of vulnerability into understandable language. Little wonder that patients resort to cliches, and poets to obscure symbolism.

Try as I might, I too am doomed when I attempt to transform subjective states into objective terminology about which everyone will have the same response. Although these four typical plights gather several types of dysphoria and disposition under a common conceptual canopy, their differences inevitably slip out from under the edges.

What these four existential plights have in common are high vulnerability, ineffective coping, and a strong concern about life and death.

Annihilation

When someone is almost overwhelmed by an amorphous dread that all is lost, any action will be futile, and the future simply cannot exist, vulnerability is enormous. Dread, anxiety, despair, and hopelessness strip everyday reality of any semblance of reliability. Values disappear; incentives are gone; familiar cues, clues, and certainties have dissolved.

There is only aloneness, which itself slips away into imminent annihilation. Such victims are bewildered as well as very anxious and apprehensive. As a rule, clinicians can only characterize such a plight as "overwhelming anxiety" or "panic reaction." Patients will say, "I am losing my mind. Who am I, anyway?"

Dread of collapse into a nameless annihilation does seem rather overdrawn. But deep within us all are traces of annihilation or what could be translated into this form of vulnerability. We do not have to be hermits to know what solitude is, nor be totally blind to imagine what it is like to grope in the dark for something we are sure is not there, nor anywhere. None of us, I trust, is wholly a stranger to dread and despair.

Annihilation is not just a matter of feeling estranged from the familiar world or even of feeling that previously accepted standards for what is real have collapsed. Authentic annihilation has such unreality and absence of self-awareness that nothing seems valid enough to be estranged from. Every statement might as well be its opposite and is not worth refuting. There are no firm convictions, no connections, and nothing can be done about it. I have known patients in whom annihilation seems so strong that they deliberately plung themselves into a fury, just to know pain and feel real again.

Anxiety is far too weak a term to cover the enormity of annihilation as an existential plight. Without a sense of reality one is wholly anonymous, another nameless, ugly face in the crowd. In the absence of time sense, the past, present, and future are only words. Because there is no change, hope is impossible.

Unworthiness belongs to demoralization and, coupled with hopelessness, further annihilates individuality. Even a maggot in a dung heap turns into a fly, and its future is assured. The wretch who is victim to annihilation feels no such promise. He is nothing at all.

I have tried to describe an extreme case of dysphoria, and we may conclude that such individuals certainly have to be crazy to feel that way. Not so, because besides knowing loneliness, unreality, and groping in the dark, one does not have to be paranoid to wonder whether people are secretly talking about us, and wish they were. Sometimes patients with advanced cancer will realize that in the course of deterioration and decline they have exchanged identities with the disease. Instead of being a person who is ill, they are now and consider themselves to be another "hopeless, terminal case." Their surplus meaning of being a sick person who has his own personality has given way or given up. Instead they become the objective meaning of a medical category called cancer mortality. They will die, of course, but before reaching that point they will have been dissolved into emptiness, spinning away into oblivion.

Alienation

I choose the term *alienation* with misgivings. It has become such a jargon word that, like *angst*, which I use later, its meaning is almost comic. The literature of alienation is enormous, and its forebears throng the pages of sociology, psychology, and many novels. Consequently, although it customarily refers to loneliness, detachment, and estrangement, the fact is that it means whatever the writer chooses, which may be a good definition after all.

From the inside, the surplus meaning is that of feeling like an exile, one who is ostracized but not as if after a specific offense, just one who feels wholly isolated, living in a kind of quarantine. Synonyms are abandonment, separation, repulsion, emptiness. The organic meaning of alienation is that of bleak separation, lack of shared meaning, living a schismatic existence.

To be alienated does not mean total solitude or independence. One can work well, fill a job with distinction, and act satisfactorily in family roles despite poverty of meaning. There seems to be no appeal or anodyne. Religion is but a distant and peculiar superstition, and in a curious way the truly alienated have a private version of God, or whatever spirit dominates the world. Such a God is ineffective, indifferent, busy with other things, and vastly overrated. Consequently, the only recourse from the abundant evil and injustice in the world is indifference. Similarly, love is a four-letter word signifying periodic sexuality. The world is over there, disavowed and hostile at best. Over here, I am deadened, depleted, indifferent to what makes other people care for each other.

That few people truly care is a grim fact that needs no further emphasis. We can learn to live with modest expectations. Although most people are afraid of loneliness, solitude can be rather pleasant. But the truly alienated go beyond solitude: there is only me, alone; you are someplace else I presume.

The alienated understand alienation. They understand that to be or not to be feels pretty much the same. When one man's hand is raised against another, to smash, not to help him up, when suffering goes unheeded because no one wants to get involved, when friends and strangers are practically identical, when people are brought together only because they share the same antipathies and distaste—all this belongs to the plight of alienation. Vulnerability is reflected in the thought, "If I were to become someone else one day, and no one noticed, well then, I might as well be nothing at all right now!" Unaffiliation is a pretty mild neologism for the ice-cold estrangement that is typical of the truly alienated. Perhaps the best phrase is *counterfeit intimacy,* that which pretends to care but is more impartial.

Endangerment

The plight of endangerment is not a simple reaction to danger. It stems from persistent frustration and inability to mobilize one's resources. When one is facing an irreversible disease or a crippling disability, the disparity between efforts to cope and progressive inability to overcome even a meager osbstacle creates blame, of self and others, combined with truculence, bitterness, and sometimes self-pity of a malignant sort.

Anger is understandable enough when there is an external obstacle that refuses to give way. What about an internal obstacle that threatens to take away existence itself? Anger at an unwelcome and unrelenting fate often leads to self-questioning doubt. "Why me?" The answer to this question, were it a genuine question, is "Why anyone?" If it were a question, instead of an entreaty, it would be an appeal for justice, as if illness and death were penalities for some unnamed crime. Fatal illness is the most impersonal fate; to ask why is simply to bemoan certainty and to resist encroachment.

If there were a formula for endangerment, it would be the following: I exist, therefore I am under siege and very vulnerable. I am angry at my fragility; I am being invaded, and my allies have deserted me.

In general, existential plights share the sense of hopeless and helpless impairment called demoralization. So too do many people who are called "neurotic." Being neurotic, insofar as this obsolete epithet means anything, refers to a state of vulnerability and being overpowered by internal forces difficult to identify and come to grips with. Some people, for example, feel helpless and oppressed by conspiratorial antisurvival forces. We call them *paranoid*. Others adopt magical strategies and superstitions as a means of finding order and reason in a world perceived as chaotic, arbitrary, and semi-insane. We call them *obsessional* and *compulsive,* because their rituals are intended to create rationality. Then there are those who are dominated by fears of the inconsequential. These are either trivial situations or exaggerations of ordinary, mundane dangers. We call such people *phobics*.

Therapists who fail to recognize the reality and urgency of existential plights are insensitive to the reality of life-and-death concerns. Or perhaps they are so concerned as to be unable to cope with their own fears of dissolution and demise. They turn instead to dubious "reconstruction" of psychogenesis, without fully understanding what brought this patient to them at that particular time. Unless therapists can see that patients bring at least a diluted version of demoralization in the form of existential vulnerability, therapy is scarcely more than a verbal fencing match between reluctant contestants. For example, patients who feel endangered may show hostile detachment, lapse into aggressive silence, use sarcasm liberally in responding to probing questions, and rebuke the therapist just for being there, because he is a potential threat.

A soft answer turneth away wrath, but a wrathful person turneth away almost everything and everyone else.

Denial

Coping strategy 15 (denying as much as possible) may not work indefinitely, and as a result, people who use it may feel anxiety, depression, and anger, along with other kinds of vulnerability. Nevertheless, in contrast to annihilation, alienation, endangerment, and encroachment, when denial is a form of vulnerability, demoralization does not seem so apparent. Patients may express outlandish and unlikely fabrications and fallacies but with a clear and disingenuous conviction that belies distress.

Now, *denial* is as legitimate as *affirmation* of a belief, and may simply be another version of a public reality with which we happen not to concur. I may deny your affirmation that the world is round or that the earth rotates around the sun, but most forms of denial are not quite that egregious. Instead they refer to topics not subject to verification because the sources of belief are private and have only surplus meaning.

After all, in ordinary life we hold opposite beliefs, conflicting opinions, divided loyalties, and contradictory notions about all sorts of things. In itself, consistency of belief has nothing much to recommend it. Without a capacity to shift grounds, change our minds, affirm and retract, or even to be steadfast, the world and its changes would be even more perplexing than it already is. Good coping needs flexibility as well as resourcefulness. If every fact known had been proved, and everything we know about were factual, there would be no reason to believe anything. Denial can be a sign of expediency that recognizes a pluralistic world and its pragmatic necessities.

Strategic negation is an essential part of objective and organic meaning. In our intrapersonal life we have little difficulty entertaining opposite ideas. Things can be relatively real and somewhat true, despite the restrictions imposed by logic. Denial helps to explain the unthinkable and tolerate the intolerable. It draws a curtain across painful facts, enabling us to live amid abundant threats.

So far, denial is both necessary and benign, hardly the stuff of vulnerability. Denial is not all bad, nor is affirmation all good. But denial of any problem and therefore of any need to cope correctly sows seeds of dismay and disaster. While language needs an instrument such as negation to clarify the uncertainties of everyday life, denial can be an expression of emotional vulnerability, too.

The most unrealistic denial of all is denial of fallibility and of certain extinction. Becker claimed that denial of death through immortality is what we endow heroes with. Gods and heroes are supposed to be immortal, of course, but they also validate our values. The combination lends absolute veracity to what we already believe. When denial takes an existential form, the individual pretends to be a god: nothing can or will go wrong. No threat exists that cannot be coped with. No doubts are tolerated.

Everything good will continue; all that is bad will dissipate. Nothing stains the pristine face of reality as it is construed.

Can we actually live with existential denial, without incurring distress and dismay of some sort? We do, just as we can live with other kinds of vulnerability. Language creates an illusion, and the illusion in turn substantiates denial. After all, unwelcome ideas are very easy to reject, and painful facts are difficult to tolerate without changing them into something else. Narcissism feeds on denial and fosters the love/hate relationship that the "I" has with itself.

The appropriate emotion that fits the existential plight of denial is *illusion*, if not self-deception. That illusion can be an emotion, as well as a misperception or mistaken belief, may seem strange to Western minds. However, contemplative minds have long accepted that illusion is a reality put there to penetrate. Things of this world are thought to be fleeting, alien, adventitious, and thoroughly unimportant compared with a higher reality that we can aspire to. This is a suprapersonal meaning that relates a person to the totality of the world, including its dreams.

Among the common coping strategies I did not include magical expectation, anticipation of miracles, or entreaties of higher spiritual forces. But there is little doubt that illusion is a widespread emotion, especially apt to show itself when we feel absolutely powerless, as in many forms of existential vulnerability. Belief in miracles or in miraculous cures is always standing by. We have only to prove ourselves the exception that will evoke the principle that stronger powers prevail. When this happens, illusion becomes the objective meaning of life, and we try to cultivate it as assiduously as possible. Serious belief in another world beyond this one, another world with reasons and resources more valid and trustworthy than those we know, will surely deny and abrogate the substance of this world, and thus do away with the painful here-and-now.

ILLUSION AND THE UNLIVED LIFE

Now I must seek indulgence in order to pursue slightly digressive fantasies that exceed the familiar scope of psychology and psychiatry. Nevertheless, I believe that the following ideas and fancies make sense out of many paradoxes that endow experience with its meaning. Thus, for me, they qualify as hypotheses.

Only objective meaning polarizes life and death into opposites. For organic meaning, living and dying are operations that are intertwined as closely as substance and shadow. Surplus meaning obviously fluctuates in its privacy between affirmation and denial, approach and avoidance, appetite and aversion, truth and illusion, being and nonbeing, living and nonliving.

From the viewpoint of these three kinds of meaning, *fear of death*, which is as close to a universal dread as we are ever likely to get, means several things: fear of extinction (objective), fear of deterioration, devaluation, and disability (organic), and fear of potential wasted or unfulfilled (surplus).

But for most people reflections about the meaning of life and death are far less frequent than ruminations about the path not taken, the "What if . . ." What if life had taken another turn; what if another option had been chosen, another door opened, another person met or married. These are old refrains, the various "might-have-beens." Such regrets and musings are well known to poets, songsters, story tellers, and just plain sentimentalists.

We know that not all fears are fears; some are wishes in disguise that we would really never act on. Other unfulfilled wishes, however, are not to be, and still seem to delineate life as it is actually lived and not just dreamed about. In this way, the path not taken helps to understand the consequences of the path we did take. Similarly, we also must realize that what we understand of the untraveled road is wholly based on the events and misadventures we actually know about directly.

I grant that much of this dream world is plain slush, woolgathering on our own time, without leading to better understanding of life as it is actually lived. A middle-aged waiter dropped out of graduate school without finishing his doctoral dissertation. He had no special training in the practical world of jobs but liked the elegance of working in fancy restaurants. He advised customers on the best dishes to order and felt very superior to his less educated co-workers. After work he gambled most of his pay, hoping for the big score that would allow him to go back to school and write his dissertation, after which he saw himself as an established authority in his field. His wife was a person of less grandiose pretensions who tolerated her husband's gambling and periodic alcohol abuse. She was convinced that her husband was "underemployed" and needed a rich father or some other deus ex machina to make things right. Otherwise, the world was unfair.

Twenty years went by, and he was no closer to his dream than ever. But his unlived life seemed to nourish and sustain him, setting him apart from other waiters who merely picked up their tips and wages. He was a loser who believed that he had other options, and in his fantasies he was a Ph.D. who happened to be a waiter.

This is a very common plight. The unlived life is lived out in the contradictory shadow of the substance. Several of Eugene O'Neill's plays have this theme. Walter Mitty also underscored his henpecked reality with heroic but unlived deeds. I can postulate that what psychoanalysts cavalierly call *reaction formations* are examples of the unlived life fueling that which is actually lived.

From an existential standpoint there are two groups of people for whom the unlived life is deadly serious. They are the potential suicides among us. One group wants to eradicate themselves completely, totally, and to be done with this world. The other group simply wants to exchange an unloved, despised portion of this life for an unlived life that is dreamed about, as constrasted with life as it is lived. Suicide is intended to get rid of the unwanted life and by partial renunciation to transform the intolerable into the ideal. Both groups visualize this life as intolerable, and the unlived life as perfect. Even oblivion is preferred.

The first group is quite serious and intent upon killing themselves along with their sorrows. But the second group will act destructively in order to search for the *illusion* that an unlived life provides. Vulnerability is enhanced by illusion. How much this influences the first and very lethal group is moot, although the ostensible reasons preceding suicide include alcohol abuse, loneliness, recent deaths of significant others, job loss, and so forth—all irremediable defects leading to despair. Perhaps the difference between these two suicidal groups is that for the second, almost any risk is worth finding the unlived but loved and elusive life. For the first, illusion has been lost; the dream has died.

Second chances are rare, and unchosen paths are usually unexplored. Although we may ruefully talk about "blessings in disguise" when justifying our lives, there are always many regrets and mistakes to ponder. It is hard to understand what makes blessings so well disguised.

Fear of potential wasted or unfulfilled is the surplus meaning of death fear. It also supplies the agony in bereavement, lost love, and vanished hopes. But fundamentally, if illusion is the emotion that sustains existential denial, *fear of death means to lose the life we never led.*

Thanatologists frequently encounter terminal cancer patients who, during a brief period of clarity prior to drifting into coma, will talk as if there is potential still unfulfilled. One woman mused about leaving her native city when her husband was transferred. She had a successful business but gave it up for his sake. Now she wondered if it were possible, after regaining her strength, to go back and start a new business.

An elderly man, following the death of his first wife, wrote to his high school sweetheart, explaining his loneliness and suggesting that they get together for a reunion, as if his unlived life could be reclaimed.

Of course, not all illusions are fictitious substitutes for the life actually lived, minus the anguish. Choices not opted for are not necessarily better, but they do tend to illuminate the substance of the choices made. In speaking with patients for the first time, whether they are medically ill or emotionally distressed, I like to ask what motivated them *at this time* to consult me or anyone else. I also look for lagging morale as well as distress and investigate past life, especially from the viewpoint of available choices made or relinquished. When did they feel best and at their best? What was it like? Looking backward, what would they like to be remembered for, what were they proudest of?

Come to think about it, I also ask these questions of myself, since they belong to the unending quest called self-exploration. By finding paired opposites in the lived and unlived life, I find that I can clarify and redefine present existence (CS 7). Actuality and illusion always need the benefit of healthy differentiation, even in the interest of honesty.

During periods of depression and alienation, it is difficult to recall times of being at one's best. Those who are threatened by annihilation anxiety, however, seem to find such questions easier to think about. "If I could only go back to when the children were young, and my husband and I had so much to live for . . ." "When I was in college and everything seemed bright, the only fear I had was that my father might die and leave us stranded." And more truculent patients tend to blame others for their not being at their best right now! Existential denial encourages the illusion that all options are open, when, in fact, such individuals are convinced at their core that no options remain.

APPROPRIATE DEATH AND THE REALITY OF ILLUSION

Many years ago, while trying to understand patients who, without qualms or questions, fully expected and accepted their own demise, I realized not only that some deaths were better than others, but that certain deaths were so fitting that they could be called *appropriate*. These were not, of course, ideal deaths, nor particularly propitious. But they did share characteristics that were consistent with good coping and sustained morale. Appropriate death, in brief, was the antithesis of suicidal death, in which an unhappy person appropriates death.

An appropriate death is one that a person is willing to claim, or even opt for, had he or she a genuine choice. It is a death to be lived with, as one's allotment and ultimate expression of being at one's best. It includes such qualities as *care, composure, communication, control, continuity,* and *closure.* What these alliterative qualities mean are the following:

Care refers to being cared for, not merely in the sense of decent medical care, but with respect to the totality of available *caritas.*

It also means caring for someone or something necessary to our morale.

Composure means to avoid extremes of emotion, even those called "positive." We cannot avoid the sadness in life or death, but vulnerability varies inversely with our capacity to cope well. Few of us are stoics, but we can learn how to contain the more vociferous and destructive dysphorias.

Communication does not mean merely to exchange words but to be able to reach a harmonious level of understanding intimacy, in which we express what we want in unambiguous terms that will be heeded.

Control is simply to recognize available options and to acknowledge that not all visualized choices are authentic. The woman who wanted to go back home and start a new business had, in her waning moments, acted as if she had an authentic choice. Not having it meant that she had lost control.

Continuity is the transition between actions that are typical of one's healthy life and those responses that recognize that potential is dwindling. Nevertheless, for an appropriate life, tokens of being at one's best can be sustained, regardless of physical plight. A dying businessman, for example, found much satisfaction when visited by his partner, who regularly discussed matters of policy as well as reminiscing about earlier days.

Closure is a matter of timeliness, when it seems just right to conclude one's business here on earth. Many people would, given a chance or, more accurately, a ghost of a chance, prefer to live on, endlessly, sharing events with their offspring and their descendants, but fortunately, this is wholly undesirable. Nevertheless, just as some people die prematurely and others live beyond any feasible significance, there is evidently a right time, a tide in the affairs of men, for embarkation.

These characteristics are not only desirable qualities for an appropriate death, but with slight variations they are entirely suitable for an appropriate life, too. I advocate the appropriate death because it is within reach of most people and their caregivers; it depends on a proper meld of reality and illusion. Features of the lived and unlived life come together as life winds down, so that reflection on what might have been and what did happen pleasantly fuse. Appropriate death is perhaps the ultimate potential to be fulfilled in the privacy of one's waning existence.

This is not a visionary or, worse, mystical approach to the inexorability of death. It is highly practical because it does not dismiss death as an illusion or a necessary evil but recognizes it for the fact and problem that it is.

Ask yourself a few questions: "If I were not what I have become, and could go back to another choice, what would I now like to be?"

"What kept me from making that choice before?"

"What prevents me from living and being something like that now?"

"Despite my failings, would I be willing to change what I am?"

"Did I really have significant options to become what I wish I were?"

"What authentic options for change do I have now?"

"Did I choose, after all, to become as I am, or was I a product of conditions beyond foresight and control?"

My digression into speculating about the value of illusion and the unlived life is now over. Although illusion has its purposes, I emphasize that self-instruction in good coping will enable most of us to make full use of our potential as long as possible, even to the doorway of death itself. It is a pretty desperate situation that leaves us with no options whatsoever. Those who feel otherwise are probably already depressed and in deep despair. A primary and prominent symptom of demoralization is to believe that because we lack a ideal option, no others are worth considering. Even a trivial option at a propitious moment is a soft declaration of control and thus may make a significant difference, just as a person who can walk away from a serious accident retains an element of choice, composure, and coping.

ANGST AND VULNERABILITY

With the same apology that I used in calling on the term *alienation*, I must take another familiar, overused word, *angst*, in order to express the dysphoria inherent in personal anguish.

Angst has no precise English synonym, but it has the advantage of familiarity as well as the problem of being used indiscriminately. It has many organic meanings, but etymology shows how provincial it is to translate the term as "anxiety." Angst covers much more. I suggest that it refers to the dysphoric range of vulnerability in its entirety.

As we contemplate the possibility of nonbeing—that is, the unthinkable potential of not existing at all—angst is what we experience. If we cannot imagine an unlived life, or a life already completed, we are woefully incomplete. Such incompleteness generates fear of fallibility (noncomprehension) and fear of faltering (noncoping). Those suffering from angst, I gather, are people who feel flawed, defective, guilty, or demoralized. In short, angst is the subjective side of vulnerability and therefore is found in many "neuroses" or "character traits." Both are recognized primarily by profound defeatism, as if there were no use trying to cope, because fate, circumstances, death, or some other self-defined misfortune makes everything futile.

PRIMARY MORALE

I have deplored demoralization, but what does morale mean? As a rule, morale is assumed to be synonymous with team spirit, solidarity, esprit de corps, common cause, and so on—whatever brings people together and unites them in a mutual enthusiasm. This is the organic meaning of morale, or as I term it, secondary morale.

Primary morale is a state of being at one's best, confident and competent enough to perform on a high level within the scope of expectable standards. It means to take responsibility for being a part of this world. The sense of confidence that primary morale inspires is the direct antithesis of angst, which fuses dysphoria of any painful kind with a disposition to fail, fall, and falter. It is quite possible to have primary morale without the reinforcement of secondary morale. This happens with pioneers who believe correctly in their cause, despite the discouragement and pessimism contributed by their contemporaries. It is also possible to have many votes of confidence but inwardly to be very shaky and apprehensive about one's competence and cause. This is secondary morale, without primary morale but with much vulnerability. As a rule, cancer patients who find themselves filled with angst can be helped by generous infusions of secondary morale. Unfortunately, the countercurrent develops when the significant care givers and friends become discouraged and drift away. When this occurs, it takes a very hardy spirit to keep primary morale from draining and becoming depleted.

Thus, the quest for morale is seldom unwavering. It reaches from the extremes of existential vulnerability to the self-confidence of coping well enough for most problems. It engages both the lived and unlived elements in life that define each other. When strong enough, primary morale can outlast and overcome the angst of vulnerability.

Perhaps morale is best understood as a belief that we can liberate ourselves from the impeding obstacles of the past and use our freedom well. To learn how best to do this, there is no alternative but to comprehend and accept consequences, without self-deception and denial. Reality may not be a Rorschach test, but its enigmas, problems, and illusions have probably been put there to see what we do with them.

CHAPTER 5

COPING, COUNTERCOPING, AND PSYCHOTHERAPY

CANCER AND PSYCHOTHERAPY

Until that day arrives, at last, when cancer can be diagnosed and cured within a short time, and treatment is readily available to anyone in need, cancer patients and others who are affected by the illness will continue to have a variety of problems to contend with. They will also need dedicated professionals and care givers with a wide range of talent, persistence, and knowledge. Their combined efforts will help strengthen such coping strategies and resources as are required for a difficult task, that of being a person who has or has had cancer.

In a curious parallel, the same predicament faces patients and families, friends and key others who are confronted with disabling psychiatric illness. Medication helps both kinds of illness, but it seldom cures. While surgical treatment is definitely out of favor in psychiatry, it remains for many cancer patients the best single modality to be offered first. Later, chemotherapy and radiation are the cancer treatments of choice, especially since choice is limited.

In cancer and psychiatric illness, coping well is mandatory. How else could we survive? Efforts to provide more or less systematic help for psychiatric patients usually include some form of psychotherapy. While cancer patients seldom opt for psychotherapy, it is obvious that help with the difficulty of coping draws on the hard-won strategies and concepts used and formulated by psychotherapists.

I used the term *countercoping* to designate the contribution that skilled and understanding care givers make to the task of coping. It complements efforts to cope insofar as good strategies are strengthened and harmful strategies minimized. The strategies used in improving how one copes with cancer and other expectable problems (Chapter 2) do not differ from those used in dealing comprehensively with so-called emotional problems in psychotherapy. There is only a shift of emphasis and extension.

Now, there are many demands put on psychiatry as it is, and I would be less than honest to claim that, despite vigor and publicity, psychotherapy has had any startling success for vast numbers of mental patients, those most in need. While I find no specific areas in cancer management where psychotherapy is particularly indicated, at the same time, basic principles of psychotherapy are unwittingly used daily in dealing with psychosocial issues that impede cancer patients.

I have combined psychiatric disability and cancer dysphorias because they are disconcerting, at the very least, and tragic, at the most. They are chronic, debilitating, demoralizing predicaments for patients and people directly involved to comprehend and cope with. In this chapter, I plan to consider the countercoping strategies that professionals and others use when they try to help people cope. How do they cope themselves? What about the wear and tear, distress, and vulnerability in a plight that tends to deteriorate or at least not to be eradicated?

In cancer and psychiatric difficulties we are also faced with existential questions. Our instruments are limited, our understanding consists largely of strong opinions, our mood is often fatalistic, and our successes comparatively few. We are challenged by failure yet sometimes overwhelmed by the challenges thrust on us.

Curiously, patients in mental (or emotional) difficulties are likely to share other characteristics with cancer patients. An unfeeling public still has antipathy, fear, and prejudice, and tends to stigmatize both psychiatric and cancer patients. Physicians who ought to know better are frequently scared by cancer patients and give up before knowing what the cancer is and whether treatment is likely to help. They have a similar attitude toward emotional distress. Some doctors are paragons of compassion, but others can be cruel and callous when confronted with chronic psychiatric disorders or with the existential shock of cancer.

To cite other parallels between cancer and psychiatric illness will not mean that there is a strong case for cancer and psychiatry. Cancer patients regularly repudiate efforts of psychiatrists and psychologists to establish an on-going relationship. "I have a cancer. I don't need a psychiatrist. It's not in my head, and I'm too busy to think about anything else. I'm only concerned about real sickness."

Although we postulate that better coping could lead to a higher morale and a better quality of life, the psychiatrist is not likely to find a receptive clientele among cancer patients. Consequently, even sophisticated physicians are unwilling to impose what they consider an additional burden. Analogously, psychiatrists who in fact seldom see physically sick people are sometimes carried away in the enthusiasm for psychodynamic explanations of cancer. Thus, they alienate patients and antagonize sources of referral. It is not unheard of for a psychiatrist to confront a cancer patient, asking what that patient has done to himself that would allow the supposed, latent anger to take such a toll.

Nevertheless, apart from what psychotherapists could or claim to do, cancer patients do have a wide range of psychosocial difficulties, some of which are distressing and need vigorous coping. What kinds of help are offered, what strategies are used, and how do these strategies compare with tactics already developed by psychotherapists?

The important differences between various theories of psychotherapy are not conceptual but entirely based on the way each persuasion defines its problems. As a result, each so-called "school" advocates certain strategies and minimizes others. For example, therapies that define problems as largely intrapsychic will emphasize formulations of conflict and find therapeutic potential in generating insight. In contrast, other schools believe that inadequacy in psychosocial situations leads to personality symptoms, such as fears, compulsions, paranoid ideas, and so forth. Their corresponding strategy is to coax or coerce reluctant patients into taking a more assertive role, to "unlearn" bad habits of withdrawal, ultracaution, and suspicion. Finally, at still another extreme, psychotropic therapists rely almost exclusively on whatever combination of medications seems likely to alleviate underlying "depression," and still profess themselves to be, in addition, good psychotherapists. When psychotherapy is minimized, it is obviously easy for anyone to aspire to and achieve the shadowy self-anointment of a qualified therapist.

Theoretical superstructures can, of course, be outlined in such detail that the onlooker believes that the differences between schools are determined by actual findings and results. I propose that different therapies use selective coping strategies for tackling problems that are themselves defined according to the strategy advocated.

Therapeutic methods are the expression of the world view of the therapist. I mean no disrespect for either patients or therapists by comparing the systems of therapy with symptoms of patients. Each is a kind of exaggeration, designed to countercope with a more or less specific malfunction.

This world view will become more apparent as I consider the relation between cancer and its psychosocial ramifications, with psychosocial methodology in general, as derived from psychotherapy. Here we shall see a link between how real problems in the outside world are coped with and the coping strategies that individual therapists use in helping patients cope.

My contention disturbs me. Are problems largely determined by the therapist's attitude, training, and experience in his own life? Is the overall purpose of therapy to persuade patients to use strategies that their therapists or other well-meaning people recommend? Do we urge people to relinquish customary interpretations of reality or of what they do in order to adopt ways and dispositions that can be coped with? The answer is, I suppose, a qualified yes. But people are often subjected to outside influence direct and indirect, the purpose of which is to change thinking and behavior. Advertising, politics, parenting, teaching, and much else have these objectives, which we tend to confuse.

It is confusing because we do not make a sharp enough distinction between benign efforts to confront, comprehend, and cope with the problems of clarifying issues for another person and the autocratic coercion that dogmatic authority seeks to impose. The first effort is to liberate people enough so that they can use autonomy well and take responsibility for being a person in their world. The second deprives a person of freedom and takes away responsibility. But in a sense autonomy and authority, as previously mentioned, make use of countercoping strategies, a situation somewhat analogous to the use we make of a hammer. It can help build a house or be a lethal murder weapon.

COUNTERCOPING AND ITS COUNTERPARTS

Coping and countercoping have a complementary relationship. Their common aim is to understand problems and to do something about them that will help. Obviously many psychosocial problems in both cancer and psychiatry are well beyond the competence of the most skilled, dedicated, and resourceful care giver. Furthermore, certain problems or concerns are so mild that strenuous efforts by highly trained professionals are superfluous, even absurd.

Intentional intervention for psychosocial purposes characterizes most efforts to intercede and change how people cope with problems reported or perceived. The plight of cancer patients who in addition to disease must deal with nonmedical ramifications may be considered typical of an existential dilemma.

The existential dilemma is not just one of living or dying but of how to evaluate what one does to lend authenticity or meaning to being alive. Cancer patients are abruptly confronted with existential dilemmas as well as many practical problems. The existential issues are, of course, frequently obscured by urgent physical and medical demands. Some investigators assert that cancer patients seem to transcend their difficulties and dilemmas by attaining a somewhat renewed appreciation of being alive and of events swirling around them. Ordinary events become extraordinary, simply because they were taken for granted for so long. Material concerns and daily struggles tend to abate and become less demanding. And so on.

I do not declare such transcendent appreciation of daily life not to exist. I am only sorry that it was not possible to go beyond material and mundane matters without becoming ill with a potentially fatal disease. But in all candor, I doubt if these transformations occur very often. The cancer plight is neither one of transcendence nor tragedy, and to romanticize the cancer "career" is to display a vast indifference to, if not denial of, the difficulties inherent to becoming gradually impaired.

At best, cancer is a heavy burden, that is borne with courage and compassion. While improvement in the quality of life will certainly enhance appreciation of everyday events, the quality of life after cancer is seldom better than it was before and is often considerably worse. Transcendence is the stuff of testimonials, not of common experience. Nevertheless, countercoping may help eliminate the more egregious and self-defeating measures that discouraged patients use in coping and defending. It is completely possible to reach an acceptable level of tolerating better what once was wholly intolerable. Then, having accomplished this modest goal, a little more may be added on.

It is possible also to magnify what care givers do, just as it is common to underestimate what is accomplished. Every interaction is not a form of coping and countercoping; this notion would be as silly as pretending that every care giver is a secret psychotherapist who attempts to rectify a psychosocial problem whenever he or she merely shares concern or gives information.

Nevertheless, just as people are seldom aware that they are speaking in sentences with punctuation, care givers are apt to offer complementary strategies in their efforts to help patients cope better. For example, responsive countercoping may take the form of advice, counseling, information, supportive services, and so on—activities that are often too ordinary to justify such a fancy designation. Just to answer a simple question may help someone cope with a nagging problem. If, for example, I cannot get out of my chair and need assistance to visit the bathroom, any help I get will be a boon and a most appreciated countercoping measure. But it is not a strategy except in a very elementary sense, because the psychosocial elements were simple.

Complementarity between coping and countercoping does not have to entail matching strategies, such as sharing concern, seeking distraction, blaming and shaming, and so forth. However, complementarity does mean that coping and countercoping are concerned about resolving the same problem and that their mutual goal is better composure, control, choice, and competence. A little help goes a long way, and a little is better than none. The countercoping I refer to here is not the comparatively trivial help offered when I mail a letter or make a telephone call. I reserve countercoping for the tasks of care givers who intentionally intervene in order to relieve distress and solve a significant problem. Countercoping counterparts also include conspicuously simple efforts, such as suggesting alternatives, encouraging independent action, directing behavior along certain lines, even jesting or offering spiritual counsel.

Care givers need to preserve morale, lest by exceeding limits or trying to do too much for too long, they exhaust themselves. Like good copers everywhere, an effective countercoper who is a thoughtful care giver will be flexible, practical, resourceful, and abundantly optimistic but only up to a point. If the left hemisphere is analytic and the right is intuitive, then both work together, and neither contribution to intentional intervention will be excluded.

Consider the following simple interchange between a cancer patient and his physician, who is about to break bad news.

DR: By the way [is this really an afterthought or what the doctor had in mind?], the X rays showed that the tumor hasn't shrunk very much, and that we [!] need more treatment. In fact, it's somewhat larger [what does this mean?]."

PT: I've already had so much treatment. How do you know that more treatment will help?

The problem is whether or not further treatment will shrink the tumor. The physician who perhaps does not even know the term "countercoping" has given information, and by saying that "we" need more treatment, he attempts to show his shared concern. The patient asks a question in response to his physician's attempt to get his consent for more treatment.

Several strategies are recognizable. Seeking information, sharing concern, redefinition, and an implication that the patient is expected to comply and conform to expectations. More accurate countercoping would spot the patient's primary problem and move in a direction that would both clarify and contain the distress that follows being informed that all previous treatment has been unavailing.

Consider another physician who must break bad news. "The tumor has definitely spread since the last time we checked it. I have other treatment to offer, but you understand that I can't guarantee anything!" Obviously, the doctor is trying to cope with his own problem, not that of his patient. His problem is how to persuade the patient to buy into a proposal that, at best, is unlikely to help, since if the treatment were any good, it would have been given earlier. Countercoping, therefore, has an inherent simplicity about a complex task. It requires just the right strategy to get a job done, without trying to accomplish too much and thereby risking demoralization and defeat.

I have used the illustration of cancer care givers because they deal with existential dilemmas. But countercoping takes place whenever a preceptor helps someone contend with a significant problem through intentional intervention. Thus, it applies to teachers, coaches, supervisors, pastors, lawyers, and anyone else who uses knowledge, enthusiasm, and trust as instruments.

TASKS AND TECHNIQUES OF COUNTERCOPING

Keep in mind that the following outline is based on complementary similarity between coping strategies and what care givers do in order to countercope effectively. Each of the following four major tasks is helped along by four types of countercoping that I call "techniques," although *technique* is hardly the best term to apply, since we are dealing with human predicaments.

1. *Clarification and control*
   Examine the problem forthrightly.
   Provide only reliable and accurate information.
   Redefine and reduce problems to manageable size.
   Consider feasibility and probable consequence of any
     action.
2. *Collaboration*
   Share concern without sharing distress.
   Refer certain problems to the respected judgment of
     another.
   Veto or prevent hasty, ill-considered actions.
   Suggest various directions and proposals that reflect
     your understanding.
3. *Directed relief*
   Encourage expression of pent-up feelings.
   Permit temporary avoidance, distraction, and respite.
   Look at familiar strategies that worked in the past.
   Allow yourself to ventilate doubt, misgivings, or con-
     fusion.
4. *Cooling off*
   Modulate and mollify tendencies to emotional ex-
     tremes.
   Encourage self-esteem and self-confidence.
   Emphasize rational, practical, prudent actions.
   At times be content to share silence and adopt a con-
     structive resignation.

Just as I specified when listing common coping strategies (Chapter 3), these are common countercoping methods and tasks that tend to be relevant for almost any problem that people try to handle by themselves. Proficient and conscientious care givers will certainly emphasize certain strategies and minimize others. Just as artists are expected to be artful, countercoping strategists are assumed to be skillful in perceiving salient problems and intervening with due respect for autonomy.

PSYCHOTHERAPY: THE UNOBTRUSIVE INTERVENTION

If I were writing a manual of psychotherapy, this would be the place to show how each coping task and countercoping technique has its special place in *my* theory of personality and practice. But before I developed my theory, I would have to admit that most practice is a mixture of improvisation, hypothesis, and deviation from these baseline procedures that I labeled "techniques."

There are, of course, many different psychotherapeutic "disciplines" and an untold number of practitioners using unstandardized, unformulated interventions that are occasionally spontaneous, often rigid and formal, and sometimes wholly opportunistic and self-serving. I do not altogether find this lamentable, because theory is completely secondary to important features of practice. Even psychoanalysts who might be expected to practice more uniformly are a diverse crowd. At times they seem to have nothing in common but a chair, a couch, and a Standard Edition.

A basic consideration in doing that specialized form of countercoping called psychotherapy is the match between patient and therapist. This does not mean that they must share a common background or that they agree on fundamental values. But there must be a basic sympathy and respect that will withstand differences in how problems are faced and formulated.

It has been claimed that responses to stress involve but a very few themes and that the therapist's personality is the key ingredient for successful intervention. If this were true, no training would be necessary, because one could be a therapist without having to learn anything more than a few simple rules of etiquette and a few more signs of impending distress. The therapist would cope in certain ways with certain patients, and cooperative patients would not be required to relinquish their own habitual strategies. Instead, they would improve what they have.

Therapists, patients, and care givers vary as much as any other group of people. There are no typical therapists, any more than there are typical parents or policemen. Personality is a factor in most vocations, but so are the predominant strategies one uses.

Therapists of quality do not have to acquire specific advanced degrees, although professional training is, I trust, mandatory. Nevertheless, I have found highly qualified therapists who were also stupid and callous, and therapists without academic degrees in counseling who seemed to have an instinct for caring well. But just as I would insist on having a well-trained surgeon perform an operation if I needed one, I also prefer that a therapist be of a certain quality.

Virtually all therapists of quality tend to listen, speak, respect, understand—assets that can hardly be argued. But they also interpret, exhort, preach, demand, prohibit, and even punish (inconspicuously for the most part), and that is by no means all, whether purists realize it or not. Therapists are known to do just about anything that one decent person with limitations and fallibilities, to say nothing of idiosyncrasies, might do for another within professional, ethical, and cultural limits. Scientific sanction is a small consideration.

Psychotherapy in practice, therefore, is shaped, limited, and directed by the training, imagination, industry, and conscience of those who make a vocation of it. Moreover, regardless of how broad-minded and nonjudgmental most therapists deem themselves, this too is a moral judgment.

Interventions in psychotherapy are not like those in regular medicine. This is an excellent reason, among others, why practitioners do not need medical training to be effective. Antibiotics, for example, are expected to be equally effective for all patients except, of course, those with specific sensitivity. And sensitivity is not related to their social class, verbal adeptness, introspective habits, or personal beliefs. But in countercoping, or interventions carried out for psychosocial purposes, these factors may be decisive in deciding which type of pyschotherapy is best suited for whom.

Because no human enterprise is absolutely objective, therapists need to work at self-knowledge as well as constantly seek to improve their repertoire of coping strategies. Enlightened self-interest is always pertinent. Part of self-interest also applies to finding out who is helped or hindered by what kinds of intervention. Some patients are prepared for verbal discourse and introspection; others are most eager for a chance to be evangelized, exhorted, or exorcised. No strategy is best.

Psychotherapists need to temper their enthusiasm or to modulate their disappointment. Regardless of the problem addressed or the procedure followed, intervention is seldom as effective as we would wish. At times resignation is the preferred strategy. But at other times not even nihilism can be counted on. However, without morale we are lost beyond redemption. Perhaps this is what redemption means: doing what has to be done to improve the competence of a lost soul.

Who elects to become a psychotherapist? There are people who manage to sway others and influence their thought and behavior just as naturally as birds fly and fish swim. A few words, a gesture, or merely their presence evokes a response that is wholly, unequivocally convincing. These are leaders who can direct thousands, and they are not apt to become psychotherapists.

Most therapists of quality differ widely, of course, but most, I believe, would settle for much less than leading hordes on a crusade. I imagine that, like most of us, therapists are willing to let someone else decide what is best, especially when problems do not concern us very much. Since we are definitely not paragons, our inclination is to be more gullible and moralistic than we like to think.

One of the occupational hazards in being a psychotherapist is identification with a fancied expert or leader. Gullibility and vacillation reach out in all directions for the certainty that independent thinking about assumptions denies us.

Demagoguery comes in many forms, often wearing a three-piece suit and surrounded by a few followers avidly insisting on their version of truth. On the other hand, a gentle manner and a soft voice are not necessarily signs of weakness or incompetence.

To hesitate a bit may mean only an effort to think a problem through before answering. A commanding presence is reassuring at times, even if the echo is louder in a hollow jar, simply because we like to be told what is right or wrong.

Many patients come to psychotherapy because autonomy has failed. Therefore, they look for direction. On their own, they are stymied and baffled. If not, then it is wise to wonder what they are doing in the therapist's office in the first place.

There can be little doubt that the single most pressing and important reason for entering psychotherapy is a sense of being demoralized. Symptoms such as fears may undermine one's sense of being in control, just as ambivalence about key relationships makes us uncertain about what to believe and how to conduct ourselves.

Demoralization is not as drastic as it sounds. For example, many people are very successful in their work and have more than adequate relationships. Still they feel constrained and incompetent, lacking the enthusiasm and belief that comes with a valid commitment to a goal. Their work provides little satisfaction, and decisions are most difficult. Demoralization among the very successful and privileged takes on a different form from the loss of self found among the very poor, the incarcerated, the obvious victims and victimizers in our society. Certain successful people begrudge themselves even a trace of satisfaction and may insist on interpreting what they do as having failed at important matters.

A young physician berated himself for establishing a highly respected but lucrative practice. He believed that were he a truly good person, he would work for free. On the other hand, had he set up practice in a very poor community, he recognized that his lack of self-regard could again lead to a reproach that he was unable to earn a good living among more exacting patients.

Blaming oneself indiscriminately is often a criterion for good or evil, as if good is whatever the individual has failed to reach or has neglected, while evil is the substance of what he has sought and attained.

Vocational demoralization may afflict psychotherapists too,

and this is not synonymous with an advanced case of burnout. Sometimes successes are so few and improvements so slight that only paradoxes and contradictions can be counted on. Being a therapist can be a lonely occupation unless one is fortunate enough to be able to share burdens without betraying confidences.

Psychotherapy *never* cures. I must be categorical, lest ambitious therapists be carried away with unrealistic expectations. As a rule, the loftier the expectation, the more uncertain the therapist actually feels. The wise and mature therapist must learn, through self-instruction, how to cope best with expectations. Conversely, it is essential to know how to avoid feeling the blame or responsibility for problems that we are unable to control, sometimes even to comprehend. Excessive expectations in the therapist leads inevitably to progressive demoralization because that therapist has not yet learned to cope with his or her uncertain plight.

Morale in psychotherapists is strengthened by maintaining composure, compassion, and controlled expectations for self and others. Am I working at my best (which is far from ideal), or do I expect too much? Am I thinking about being able to do more than actually can be accomplished? If I were my patient, what would I expect, and how reasonable is that?

Many psychotherapies founder when therapeutic ambition is too great. True enough, highly touted methods have earned much money for their advocates. But because follow-up evaluation is lacking for *any* method, we can hardly believe that fads and financial gain prove the worth of what is advertised to be effective. The more grandiose methods, therefore, are most suspect.

Psychotherapy can, however, mitigate misery and maybe help establish a stronger sense of morale. This seems like a very modest goal, especially when one considers the exaggerated claims that various schools and persuasions foster. Few people are satisfied because most believe that a little more might have been accomplished. Yet this is often more than enough to permit a patient to take a place again in his or her psychosocial stratum with confidence and competence, willing even to assume responsibility for being a part of the world.

Obviously, I am against the psychotherapeutic hustle promulgated by professional pitchmen. Patients largely succeed by themselves, with only the indirect help of an understanding and unobtrusive therapist. Few therapists of quality cast themselves in the role of sorcerer, shaman, guru, or magician.

I can entertain the image of a miraculous healer who touches and treats, cures and confers great enlightenment. It would be glorious to be in the presence of an infallible sage or leader who would anoint me, of course. He should not only be thoroughly conversant with all the ills that beset mankind but have names for them and solutions. This image even goes beyond the apotheosis that many patients have for their surgeon.

My realistic vision of a capable psychotherapist of quality is one who provides quietly unobtrusive countercoping. If, however, such a practitioner has substantial autonomy of his own and believes it indispensable for patients to acquire a more profound sense of their own responsibility in coping well enough, then his influence will be almost as powerful as if he were really able to intercede with preternatural forces. The therapist of quality makes no holistic profession, but he appeals to undeveloped and unrecognized qualities in the patient. He disavows exaggerated expectations and demands, whether coming from himself or others. He is no listening post for truth, nor a model for anyone to emulate. Nevertheless, like most ostensibly simple people, he—or she—is as complicated as anyone else.

More specifically, what does an unobtrusive practitioner do? Even with manifold fallibility, idiosyncrasies, and limited repertoire, such a therapist of quality attempts much more and his interventions are far more elaborate than is apparent on the surface.

In the previous section, I listed a few of the more prominent tasks and techniques of countercoping. Here are other ways in which unobtrusive interventions carry out the aims of better morale, along with strategies for countercoping.

    (1) Collaboration (with another person)
    (2) Comprehension (of another)

(3) Clarification (for oneself)
(4) Composure (for oneself and another)
(5) Relief (of another's distress)
(6) Decision (for oneself)
(7) Choice and control (for another)
(8) Reward (for oneself)
(9) Hope and trust (for another)
(10) Respect and regard (for oneself)

Glancing over this somber list of interventions, a reader would be justified in wondering who is being helped to cope, the putative therapist or the presumed patient? I suggest that both are helped in different ways. Helping another person to cope better and develop stronger autonomy can certainly benefit the counter-coper, just as a piece of music is improved by the integrated contributions of theme and counterthemes, melody and counterpoint.

If we were to put aside the medical model—or the evangelical model, for that matter—what remains is an interaction between two people, at least one of whom has trouble maintaining a decent level of morale. While the formal doctor-patient relationship is presumed to have a therapeutic aim and value, interaction or confrontation between people meeting because of an existential dilemma has a seamless mutuality.

Comprehending, collaborating, clarifying, making decisions, encouraging options, offering selective support, and so on, are distinct elements of countercoping that come together and fuse.

When the transaction goes well, tasks and techniques, ends and means, outcomes and strategies are indistinguishable. For example, if I want information and ask someone for it and get it, then asking and receiving are the same. But when all does not go well, the transaction splits into different parts, causing varying amounts of distress. The unobtrusive therapist may be blamed for not being active and assertive enough, or for being unwittingly intrusive! The therapist can be idealized upward and downward, from an angelic position to the devil incarnate. But as a rule, negative responses to countercoping are fairly temporary and can be clarified along with restoring composure, allowing for the patient's relief, and going on to making professional decisions that will amplify the patient's opportunity to choose and to control.

The agenda of unobtrusive interventions depends on a reasonably harmonious meeting of minds. We expect a certain amount of flexibility as well as rigidity in both participants, because undue passivity or unyielding superiority, if both occur at once, leads only to conversion of the faithful.

Anger benefits no one; it only demonstrates poverty of strategic responses and perhaps can be fatal to a successful termination in mutual respect and regard or hope and trust. Unobtrusive interventions require respect and trust, regardless of what else happens during therapy. And if these can be encouraged, morale may revivified enough to endure.

The quality of hope is hoped for, just as we trust that we encourage trusting attitudes. But mere hope for a positive change is not enough to guarantee that change. If, for example, I hope for a remission of cancer, I can expect it or not, but my biology will have the very last say. Vulnerability may outlast our pious hopes. Indeed, self-deception thrives on counterfeit hope. Authentic hope is based on doing something that will strengthen autonomy and competence, ultimately self-esteem. Counterfeit hope exploits sickness, leading us to pine away, yearning for the unattainable. The unobtrusive therapist with ample morale embodies authentic hope, but the huckster sells counterfeit hope along with his snake oil.

While psychotherapy works, most conscientious therapists readily acknowledge that it does not work nearly well enough or often enough. Nevertheless, to be sustained by down-to-earth expectations means that hope is tempered by realistic trust in someone else's fallibilities and good faith. We are certainly limited in almost every direction. But limitation is not equivalent to being afraid of falling, faltering, failing. Angst is only a trace element in unobtrusive countercoping. This is not to advocate a cocksure arrogance. Overconfidence in a therapist is like entitlement in a patient. Both are duplicitous, manipulative, and hypocritical. They mean bad faith and pseudomorale.

ENCOUNTER, EMPATHY, AND FAILURE

Every intercession presupposes an encounter in which one person meets another at a moment of need and resolves to undertake a mutual task of clarifying and understanding that need. But the presupposition embodied in psychotherapy is that failure of autonomy has brought about demoralization, depletion, and a sense of defeat. Furthermore, it is expected that need translates into want and that the want becomes a valid expectation. Moreover, because competence and integrity are assumed, the prospective patient yearns for and then relies on the other person to fulfill what is usually quite unrealistic, far-fetched, and unlikely.

Theoretically, intentional intercession for therapeutic purposes can take place anywhere, any time, except that it seldom does. Merely to come together is nothing more than bumping into another person. Even if the other person is well-intentioned, sober-minded, and very attached, there is no assurance that needs will be recognized or responded to. For example, few people know how to respond when confronted with someone in the throes of acute mourning after death of a loved person. Coming together with the mourner may be an occasion of acute embarrassment, if not one of faltering and failing to respond constructively in this encounter. As a result, people tend to talk about everything and nothing, just as a mourner listens to everyone and nobody. People struggle to console, support, explain, and justify—all of which is wholly inappropriate and somewhat offensive. "I think your father wanted to die," "Her suffering is over," "It must be God's will," "Death is a part of life, and we must realize that life goes on." I could multiply these inanities indefinitely. There can be a babel of silence, or of sounds because words can mean less than silence. If an encounter with an existential dilemma consists of nothingness, customary talk at the place of sadness and bereavement represents absurdity and helplessness, especially in those who would help if they could.

At the opposite end of the existential encounter that clarifies nothing, where dumb sympathy and confused talk try to turn loss into a kind of achievement, is the classic example of a Socratic dialogue. Because it is very rational, verbal, and conducted in a spirit of inquiry about a lofty topic, the dialogue presupposes the importance of discourse, reasoning, and mutual perception. Proof and demonstration are assumed to be sufficient to change anyone's mind. There is love of wisdom and truth; this is about the only emotion permitted. Life and death crises or existential dilemmas are as remote as the sun. Actually, apart from their portentous subjects, Socratic dialogues convey the feeling that nothing much is at stake.

On the face of it, Socrates professed ignorance and ostensibly questioned others, seeking knowledge and understanding. To do so, he asked others to instruct him. He countercoped, clarified, collaborated in a quest for enlightenment.

The Socratic method has become the beacon of detached pursuit of truth, even though Socrates' persistence disclosed that he was well aware of where he was going and what he believed. But he did think that everyone had an innate knowledge of truth and that ignorance was only a veil that could be lifted by self-examination with the help of others.

Psychotherapy is situated somewhere between the detachment of Socrates and the baffled confrontation with enigmas of life and death. The story of Job is too well known to recount here, but no one had an answer for Job, and it was difficult to help him cope with misfortunes and tragedies. If we wanted in some anachronistic way to countercope with Job, what would we do? How much responsibility and reason could be imparted to a meaningless, horrendous plight? What meaning could be conveyed? That is what Job wanted to know. How best to help Job cope without trying to rationalize his plight? What if we were his psychotherapist? What would be asked of us, or what might we ask of ourselves? The therapist of quality is not ashamed to acknowledge ignorance, innocence, or inadequacy. He knows the value of silence, and the importance of being sensitive to specific needs, some of which can be relied on, while other professed needs are spurious.

If I were Job's psychotherapist, perhaps even his friend, I would silently register my feeling *for* his plight, without pretending that I knew *exactly* how he felt. Obviously, I could not answer what was in God's mind when he chose Job or why God tried to match wits with the forces of evil. But after awhile I would ask Job what he saw ahead of him, what one practical thing he might do now, considering everything that had happened. As the acute distress abated, I should also assess and evaluate Job's options, find out how he coped with other difficulties in the past, and then support through alliance and further inquiry his efforts to cope now. I would not try to explain, justify, or otherwise obfuscate by pretending to understand more than I had—nor less, for that matter.

A good countercoper needs to be less vulnerable than the person attempting to cope, but he is no stranger to vulnerability. The psychotherapist of quality needs to use both sides of the brain, in that analysis and empathy share in the authentic encounter. These are polar opposites, of course, as represented by the classic Socratic dialogue and the wordless compassion for suffering we experience in the presence of mourning.

Turning to the imponderable question of empathy, I acknowledge its value, of course, but find it hard to assay. Buie sagely pointed out that empathy can be overrated and mistaken, especially when a therapist infers too much from meager cues, or for that matter, from practically no cues at all. We are all fallible, but the major flaw in some therapists is that they do not recognize their fallibility; they assume that if an idea or insight occurs to them, it must therefore have a basis in the patient's mind. There is always a hidden temptation to attribute thoughts to another person that simply are inaccurate. As previously pointed out (Chapter 4), we can share objective meanings of words but differ widely as to their organic meaning and, of course, their surplus meaning.

Alienation is triggered by lack of trust and respect, and in my opinion, empathy is impossible without trust and respect for another. Like a love that cools down, once alienation has occurred, reconciliation and renewed affiliation are very difficult. Of course, the therapeutic affiliation is not at all like being in love, fortunately; but empathy, when authentic, seems to generate much more trust and respect for another person than occurs in an infatuation.

The tasks of countercoping are never clearer than when therapist and patient join together in understanding their differences and sharpening their mutual perception of meanings. Empathy will not only tolerate differences but there is an authentic *desire* to see the world through another person's eyes. Clearly, an overly intellectual approach to psychotherapy puts a distance between patient and therapist, while an excessively emotional attitude is apt to become maudlin or, in some cases, frightening to both parties.

A good therapist, therefore, cultivates a capacity to appreciate other kinds of values besides his own; he understands how another person defines a successful act. As a result, empathic understanding comprehends the nature of success and feels for the person who is afraid of faltering and losing self-esteem. If interpersonal resonance is reasonably clear, the therapist knows how the patients copes and defends, suffers and feels good.

But it is also reasonable to wonder what makes empathy valuable, if indeed it does serve a therapeutic purpose. Maybe empathy is nothing more than misplaced enthusiasm for our own surmises, just as, for example, listeners can impute arcane and subtle meanings to a piece of music that were, presumably, never intended by the composer.

Most of life's situations do not call for a high titer of empathy. Moreover, the quality of being empathic has been exaggerated in certain circles, as if it were a sign of a fine character that could stand by itself, without the corrective influence of analysis.

As a therapist, and in the privacy of myself, I shuttle between rationality and ill-formed emotion, knowing that the distinction between them is largely one of emphasis. For me, empathy means *respect for another person's irrationality.* If I can also trust another person, despite irrationality, then empathy has its own organic meaning, which is not a special gift for looking behind the mental scene into another person's private theater.

Using this definition, empathy can be learned, even taught. The first lesson, however, consists of knowing that nodding one's head sympathetically, and saying, "I understand exactly how you feel," means nothing more than "How I feel is the way I expect you to feel."

Participating in another person's world means a *desire* to see the world through his or her eyes; it does not mean sharing another person's experience, because that is impossible. If it *were* possible, then several times every day I would laugh or cry, be angry or indifferent, feel anxious or sad, with feelings utterly not my own.

To have empathy seems to have a special value all its own, a gift possessed, not altogether unlike clairvoyance. Whenever I hear some passionate champion of empathy eloquently declaiming his sensitivity by stating that there is no crime he could not have committed, though he may never have had a traffic ticket, I am sure that it is not empathy for the criminal he professes. Rather, it is his own unlived lives, perhaps his criminality in contrast to being meticulously law-abiding, that he imagines, plus, of course, a large dose of dramatic license. Respect for a real person's irrationality does not seem to belong to this type of flamboyant expression. Since it is a quiet talent, and one that can be learned, empathy of the respectful kind is likely to be found in the unobtrusive therapist.

I cannot really feel another person's pain and do not believe others when they claim to. Even if I tried very hard, I could no more wince at your pain than I could be convinced of your delusion. But I do and feel much that has no tangible basis, except as my private disposition. Nevertheless when I hope, fear, yearn, or am repelled, trusting, and withdrawing from—a vast array of feeling—these active sentiments sometimes seem to provide a peephole into existence. Even common feelings can estrange us. It is not unusual suddenly to feel, even among friends and associates, that we are all strangers speaking an alien tongue we are familiar with. Nothing seems to be communicated; no one understands, yet no one shows it. But perhaps strangers trust and respect us, despite our differences, and for ordinary purposes empathy is irrelevant. The psychotherapist of quality does not concern himself with whether or not he possesses that rare gift of empathy in its arcane sense. But being prepared to trust and respect another person, he hypothesizes about motives and meanings. "I would not have done that, or said what he did. What prompted him to act that way? The reasons he gives me are not very convincing. Besides, they come to his lips too readily. He makes sense, but I can't make sense out of him. Let me just take him on his terms for a moment. What would it be like to be in that kind of situation? How much of what I feel would be the right thing in his place?''

Self-instruction makes use of error and fallacious surmise. It deals much with paradox; namely, understanding how two or more truths that seem incompatible are not. If I make an outrageous statement, such as, ''The only people who should be permitted to pray are atheists,'' everything about the remark seems senseless. Atheists don't pray; permission to pray is not something to be granted; and prayer is a distinct privilege of religious people. These are three apparent truths that are combined in a paradox. The paradox is useful, however, if it refers to three different meanings of the statements that are condensed into a fallacious remark that could easily offend everyone, atheists and the religious alike.

I imagine that the only time an atheist could be induced to pray to a god he doesn't believe in is when it is forbidden, or when he is sufficiently desperate to try anything. Suppose also that the religious could be forbidden to pray on the grounds that *not* to pray is a test of faith somewhat comparable to asking an atheist to pray and thereby test his nihilism on the firing line, so to speak. Finally, when I give permission to pray or refrain from prayer, I take on a hypothetical task of comparing one person's convictions with another's. Which will be sturdier and more resistant—the believer or nonbeliever?

Paradox represents a failure to empathize correctly, because when the apparent inconsistency is understood, a curious sense of validity emerges. Failure means to falter in efforts to comprehend and cope. This is a common enough event among psychotherapists. Failure can, however, be a source of learning, as every schoolboy is taught, and success is a product of finding ways to justify our values.

I surmise that in its more unobtrusive moments psychotherapy is a compassionate exercise in finding the beneficial use of failure so that demoralization can be overcome. And failure may be the result of not understanding certain basic paradoxes. Unraveling a paradox is one of the most instructive ways of developing empathy. But empathy does not mean empty echoes of our own guesses. Compassion, trust, and respect do not require absolution, agreement, or advocacy. Success is, of course, rewarding, but failure also has potential for self-instruction. Such is the therapist's plight, however, that he can never be quite sure, since certainty is not to be trusted. Please think about *that* paradox.

THE THERAPIST'S CONSOLATION

Having prepared the reader for paradoxes, it will be understood when I claim that psychotherapy is either very easy or practically impossible. That is why poorly trained counselors do well, and their results are scarcely different from the most highly experienced practitioners. Few other fields can make that claim. The mystique and pseudoscience surrounding the art and practice of psychotherapy cannot obscure the fact that results are largely anecdotal.

I suppose that an elderly teacher might have similar reflections at the end of his career. Despite utmost dedication, combined with knowing much about his field, and deriving ample rewards and recognition, he cannot be sure of what he has accomplished. After all, good students might have learned as much from any teacher, and poor students left his classes scarcely better than when they began.

Psychotherapists, too, must recognize the disparity between their efforts and results. They need protection against a sense of failure that is bred from expecting too much. Therapists with very lofty ambitions are usually those who are spurred by a sense of weakness and incommensurate pride. No worthwhile therapist who takes his job seriously is without moments of doubt and demoralization. That, after all, is what coping and vulnerability are about. There are painful times when a creeping nihilism takes over, causing a therapist to think that he is either a mountebank offering nothing but vain hopes, or an entrepeneur trading on misfortune and gullibility.

A professional should be able to tolerate, even learn from failure. He must distinguish between what is obvious, likely, possible, probable, and totally out of the question. He is paid to do a competent job, not to promise to do the unlikely or to perform miracles.

Those who belong to the so-called helping professions should realize that they are being helped too. Any profession can be called "helping," and it is only because mental health professionals question their intrinsic value that they single themselves out for this designation.

True professionals, in the sense of being a psychotherapist of quality, know how to cope and to countercope. These are skills they learn through self-instruction. Its major aim is to rescue therapists from overweening pride or overwhelming futility. Quality control in psychotherapy is largely internal, where the critic has an investment in the performer.

The key quality that enables a conscientious therapist to go on unobtrusively is the capacity to cope with ambiguity. Coping is not only necessary, along with skill and empathy, but the therapist must understand what can reasonably be hoped for, so that he can disavow the rest, regardless of what others try to thrust upon him.

Unobtrusive interventions are what count, because their purpose is to help patients develop skill, empathy, morale, and self-esteem. Unobtrusive interventions require unobtrusive expectations. This is a coping skill that counteracts undue pride and self-deception.

I have already asserted that psychotherapy and counseling may suffer from its own extravagant expectations. Bombastic terms, such as rebirth, transcendence, actualization, are slogans intended to promise much more than can be imagined, except during heights of rapture about a future that will never come. I do not object to those who would rise above ordinary humanity for protracted periods. After all, this should not be very difficult, considering the low standards that most people have. I am, however, cautious about panaceas. I close my ears to bugles announcing not only that the psychological millenium has arrived but is coming down the street.

Unobtrusive countercoping is like steady, good coping; neither is very conspicuous, even to the person who carries them out. It takes a very bitter therapist, or patient, for that matter, to deny that certain changes for the better do occur occasionally during therapy. Positive gains do happen, although encounters are far from complete, methods are crude and inadequate, disappointment is frequent, and prediction very uncertain, as it is in human affairs.

The unobtrusive therapist usually finds his rewards equally modest and quiet, as testimonials go. Reports of great success are likely to be exaggerated downward into subdued gratitude.

We can turn back to management of the dilemma called cancer mortality and inexorable disease. Any of us would like to spare patients pain, disability, dysphoria, and every other expectable and distressing problem. We also seek a therapeutic resource that is sure, unerring, brief, and within the reach of all. If necessary, such management must be miraculous. Fantasy, obviously, need not suffer restriction.

Psychotherapists of quality know that lofty aspiration is most poignant when suffering is most intractable. Cancer and psychological anguish meet in common cause. I am told that St. Jude is the patron saint of lost causes, whether cancer or impossible psychosocial problems. Therapists have no saints to monitor our lost causes, nor to measure the inadequacy of our competence. However, when respect and trust combine with courage and compassion, they begin to mean something. The combination adds substance to the endeavor.

Therapists need skepticism in the way that a traveler needs immunization. A naive therapist, filled with enthusiasm and book-learning, might wander the face of the earth, looking for a messianic message about mankind. He would be compassionately understood if he listened to guides who claim too much, too loudly. His travels will find him turning this way, then that way, learning much, and a lot that is misleading. If he pledges loyalty first to this school, then to that method, professing now one set of values, then forsaking them for another, finally he will have nothing to show for his efforts but battered baggage.

If a psychotherapist of quality needs consolation, he must be able to cope with blind alleys and intriguing byways as well as with major obstacles. Coping well enough, without exaggerating his potential, should be emblematic for the therapist. Self-exploration is never complete; autonomy is always conditional. Unobtrusive interventions often will leave something substantial for the therapist. Perhaps the consolation that is most substantial is perseverance. This is an assurance of more than adequate morale, which bestows a great favor for the unobtrusive therapist: not to need consolation.

CHAPTER 6

THE TEN-SPEED
LIFE CYCLE

Unfortunately, those who learn to cope best do not necessarily live longer, or even die better deaths. Unexpected events are always intruding. Nevertheless, it is quite possible that they have also learned how to sustain morale, and therefore, with a little luck, achieve a better quality of life that will not endanger them.

Because existence is so evanescent, aging is a universal metaphor for things that come into being and pass away. This is one of the world's oldest philosophical problems. It also characterizes what we understand about all organic life.

In previous chapters I have emphasized coping strategies that can be identified and dealt with as they occur and recur. There are also *longitudinal channels* in the course of life that contain and direct different forms of conduct and problems. These too constitute different perspectives on coping because they are parts of the life cycle, as it is customarily called. Each part, which I shall call a *subcycle*, is expected to work well with the other components, not just to endure but to articulate in a common task and thus to arrive by distinct paths, more or less together, at a distant point, *old age*.

With this perspective I intend to reverse the usual custom of starting at the beginning. Instead, I prefer to visualize the course of each subcycle from the retrospective standpoint of old age, looking backward to see if any general principles can be discerned. This seems like a fitting procedure, since if all works well, every subcycle will ultimately be brought to a penultimate focus. As a rule, when beginning at earlier phases, investigators are forced, even against their will, to surmise about the causative effect of prior events on the fate of the future. Since no one can actually do this, they borrow from what they already know, peeking at the back of the book, and then trim their versions of childhood and adolescence with the understanding given by middle and old age. This results not just in a "soft determinism" but in a spuriously dogmatic framework in which one set of events substantively predisposes to another. Plights and problems, like people, differ in almost every conceivable way with the passage of years. The so-called "genetic viewpoint" is woefully unable to comprehend the sequence of how things come to be as they are, unless later events are projected backward into hindsight. It is correct to note that almost anything can happen to almost anyone, but to some more often than others. Every culture has its own mythology, including the story of creation and how the world comes to an end.

I have already observed that certain eras cast shadows across themselves with prototypical diseases that typify the times. It is not insignificant that these diseases are all associated with inevitable death, without exception, and that a strong element of ostracism precedes death. Our modern scene views old age in much the same way as it does cancer mortality. The decay of senility is as frightening as the intractable pain dreaded in advanced cancer. One man, for example, was relieved to learn he had pancreatic cancer. He had feared living long enough to become as helpless and senile as his father who spent many years in a nursing home because of dementia. A dignified death in the near future was more welcome.

We also must remember that aged people are just as likely to retain the same beliefs about old age as they held when young. Disability, dementia, poverty, erosion of spirit and body, fear of death and its depredations—all these are familiar spectral visions and very bleak realities for some. Aging is a metaphor for loss of almost everything held to be worthwhile, from loss of youth, glamorized beyond fact, to deterioration of mental acuity. Euphemisms about the "golden years" are hypocritical; otherwise, no euphemisms would be required.

The comparison between old age and cancer mortality is by no means far-fetched. Aside from hypocritical euphemisms, the aged are told about their wisdom but also advised to relinquish and renounce what is no longer theirs to choose, as if they suffered from a chronic malady that has no cure and very little palliation.

Old age has, even at best, a kind of monotonous melancholy that differs sharply from the high hopes and expectations given to younger people, illusory or not. After all, there is just so much and so little time. Meanwhile, being older reminds us that mankind is infinitely replacing itself. Nevertheless, there is a clear difference between being transient and being replaceable. The latter is generated by a throw-away mentality that saps morale as well as vitality. Transience has its own value. It treasures the moment, epitomizing the worth of the person who is now here, but then passes into memory.

Assuming that one possesses a healthy measure of physical and mental integrity, awareness of death as a necessary event, not a remote speculation, puts a fine edge on being alive. It certainly gets our attention, anyway. Morale can be low at any age. The ebb and flow of competence and confidence take place throughout the drifting toward extinction we call the course of life.

Only the young can afford to think about immortality. The very old realize that the promise of an unlimited future has many conditions and perhaps is an empty offer after all. Not only is old age a period of misgivings for one's competence and morale, but it is often a time of conspiracy in which every function seems to slow down. Nevertheless, it is still useful to distinguish between the vigorous who are old and the decrepit who suffer most from the inroads of senescence.

While I do not minimize the risks and reality in growing older, there is no point to deploring it. The aging process has many components, just as the life cycle has many subcycles that run at their own speed, in separate directions, for different purposes. Not all diminish, falter, or fail. Special problems and coping strategies differentiate one subcycle from another, and these help to individualize one person from another.

I advocate an even-visioned appraisal of what growing older means, using the different kinds of meaning described earlier (Chapter 4). Aging is not a series of uniform or homogeneous events. For some, growing older actually may turn out to be the vintage years, while for others the wine is very bitter indeed. Aging does have the chill of certain death, but it is not the ague of sickness, merely the melancholy of passing away. Coping strategies may become very limited, but choices are still there. Newer challenges appear, to be met with appropriate guidelines.

WHAT MAKES THE LIFE CYCLE CIRCULAR?

Aging is not only a universal metaphor but its imagery has been caught up in our thinking, as if the time from birth to death bends back on itself, almost touching. Pedants think about life cycles, and life cycles are typical of how pedants think. There are many things shared and perpetuated from youth through old age. No special segment has exclusive rights to any thought or feeling. Pedants conceptualize the life cycle into divisions called stages, phases, species, generations, and so on, but nature does not behave so methodically.

We do know, of course, that youth is not the same as old age, and that except for the metaphor of ashes to ashes, we never return to the stage of the past. We do not resume infancy, adolescence, and middle age. Life cycles are not therefore very circular; other images are just as plausible—a spiral, an arrow, a hyperbole, a pool of water, and so on.

For me, the life cycle is more like a ten-speed bicycle. A bicycle seems so simple and silent, self-propelled and sufficient. The rider with skill does not fall, but even the expert can meet with an accident or be struck by an unanticipated lethal force. Wheels within wheels, pulleys, clamps, wires, and bolts are fastened to-gether to give the rider an illusion that he is wholly in control. Furthermore, given a good instrument to begin with, the rider comes to believe that he and his bicycle are one, and that the terrain is not at all hostile or unpredictable. At that point, he has taken too much for granted. He forgets, for example, that it is only by moving ahead that he keeps from falling off. He is very dependent on even minor attachments. His attention cannot waver; the consequences of his action may catch up in the next moment. He copes and hopes so frequently that habit and skill become second nature, and he never retraces his path in exactly the same way.

Enough of this metaphor. No one knows who invented the wheel but it is certainly a substantial part of how we think about the world and our place in it. Part of the reason I favor that version of the wheel called the ten-speed bicycle is not only to find a place for subcycles but to emphasize that smooth coping with potential problems may lull a complacent rider into believing that risks and accidents are negligible. Only the rider repeats himself; the wheel is not absolutely circular and does not return to its beginning and start over. We need more than a good machine to cope well enough.

The extremes of birth and death are close to total opposites in both a biological and cultural sense. Customarily, birth is celebra-ted, death is mourned—but not necessarily. Another face to feed and a beloved elder dead, and the custom is reversed. But for the most part, whatever begins at birth belongs to the inception of a journey that carries traces into the future. The exact path cannot be planned in advance, because each subcycle, with subsidiary sub-subcycles, has its own program.

TEN SUBCYCLES TO COPE WITH

Here is a list of ten subcycles, essential to a larger life cycle, which, activated at birth, express themselves in different ways until they finally come together at or near the time of death.

(1) Chronological uniformity amid change.
(2) Developmental interaction
(3) Physical well-being and health
(4) Psychosocial adaptation
(5) Psychosexual fulfillment
(6) Racial, ethnic, cultural and tribal et ceteras
(7) Ideological affiliations
(8) Personal and mental distinction
(9) Politico-economic deployment
(10) Thanatologic realization

Chronological uniformity amid change

As a concept, time scarcely measures anything except change. For instance, it does not measure endurance, persistence, even duration of illness. This moment, that you and I share, is both ancient and new. It is gathered from the centuries and from our mutual past. Inwardly, I recognize traces of my childhood and later life, brought somehow to a focus. I assume the same for you, and as a result of different changes, we probably share only this moment in its objective meaning.

Many layers of past events support each other, just as the ground we stand on is supported by other eras. Chronology varies with the order of magnitude of events filling it with change. Therefore, how old anyone is cannot wholly be a matter of time elapsed since birth according to a calendar. Age is arbitrary to some extent, because rocks have an age, mayflies age, trees age, living organisms age, and even inanimate objects age, insofar as they change.

What does the measuring stick of age measure, besides itself? Chronology is a conceptual convenience that establishes uniformity amid change. Subcycles have their own variable speeds, rate of change, and intrinsic events that determine changes. Standard deviations are somewhat unknown, except for the biological differences between old and young, and from one person, old or young, to another. I am older or younger than you, only according to one or another subcycle, or perhaps all of them collectively. Conversely, if elapsed time had a distinct and separate reality, the concept of a life cycle would be as meaningless as an empty space. Events and their sense of reality, which means simply the events that matter most, decide what events are decisive, and therefore what time elapsed really signifies. We are simultaneously old and young, depending on the use we make of abstractions. Time is like a thread along which we string some beads.

Developmental interaction

Under this heading I must include everything that pertains to growth, maturation, size, and function relating to organs, body parts, and workings thereof, from microscopic genes to a fully developed *homo sapiens.*

The brain grows and folds during early development, keyed by factors and forces still being investigated and named. The newborn does a number of remarkable things that fetal life anticipates, but it takes awhile before anyone climbs trees, learns languages, operates machinery, and observes himself doing all this and more and wonders about it. Of course, the brain does not do this by itself. It is an organ central to healthy developmental interaction of every other organic part with distinct and manifold functions.

Developmental interactions are most prominent early in the life cycle. Healthy interactions provide the organic basis for what is the substructure of coping. Other subcycles are initiated later. For example, ideological affiliations and politico-economic deployment need a more secure organic base, combined with the capacity to know languages and use symbols. Evolution apparently sees to it that growth and development occur rather rapidly at first to safeguard survival, although most organisms are independent more promptly than the human. But that is a matter of relative coping potential and the kinds of tasks that men and women cope with.

Development takes many curious turns, especially as other subcycles become more prominent. For example, growth and development are early starters among subcycles in order to assure survival, but extended dependence is a psychosocial force that also protects the young. However, cultural and social customs ultimately decide who is to become an adult and acquire the restrictions and obligations special to that clan or tribe.

Protection of the young and safeguards for survival are not always for the sake of the child. A child may pick grapes, sweep floors from morning until night, wash dishes, and empty slop buckets. Despite being treated as a somewhat helpless semiadult, the child is deprived of more complete growth and maturation. Organic interaction will be impaired as much and as fully as a child kept from learning is an aberration denied full growth. Neglect stunts maturation by exploiting physical developmental interaction.

Physical well-being and health

There is no formula that provides an absolute guide for physical well-being and health throughout the life cycle. If there were, such a formula would be far more precious than any other acquisition and commodity, since without health everything else withers.

Thus far, except for a few genetic disorders, medical science has not been able to tag those at greatest risk for specific maladies. There are too many aberrant factors that intervene and spoil most attempts to find a simple formulation. Holistic medicine, as it is currently called, is an ancient art, recurrently rediscovered. It is based on the idea that disease is preventable by fully using man's capacity to cope with and even change his propensity to fall ill. But how this remarkable concept is implemented remains quite obscure. It is far easier to provide testimonials and to make heated declarations than to offer specific strategies.

Health principles are not the reverse of a deleterious life style filled with harmful habits. The wages of sin, so to speak, may be fatal, but the wages of virtue are uncertain. No one is spared illness, ailments, and disease, and old age is elastic enough to include the healthy and the decrepit. The subcycle of physical well-being is undermined in various ways, so that the chronologic young can be quite elderly. We like to believe in holistic medicine because it gives us a hypothetical opportunity to participate in our own welfare and therefore to cope with threats to health. It is even a moralistic cause, implying that a set of healthy habits can postpone the aging process. Those who are ashamed of growing older often seek a cosmetic rejuvenation, if not a chronologic reversal. Many people would gladly change places with Dorian Gray. Inevitable illnesses supervene anyway, and in some older people the painful journey toward limbo results in devaluation as well as decline. But prejudice against the aged exacts penalty, too. Suppose, for instance, there were a society in which old age was honored and became more esteemed as years went by. A slight stoop, a halting gait, a wrinkled face, and lessened stamina might be chic, in just the way that a deep suntan suggests much leisure and considerable affluence.

But old age does not automatically ensure distinction, and even the distinctive become obsolete. Physical appearance of age is almost a stigma, and cosmetics sell better than exercise equipment. Nevertheless, physical health and well-being is a subcycle that emerges from chronology and developmental interaction. It requires acquisition and maintenance of health habits. This does not merely refer to adequate nutrition, avoidance of toxic substances, and exercise programs. Healthy coping strategies spread out over time are better called skills, practices, and customs that contribute to well-being and physical health. Healthy customs become a way of life, not a program, but collectively there are ways to cope with implicitly deleterious tactics that undermine health and well-being. This subcycle continues throughout life, and is as relevant for the inactive older person as for the vigorous teenager. Problems are apt to change as time goes on. A hearty good fellow who holds his liquor well in college may lose everything else later in life, and this includes his liver.

There is an art to anticipating and solving problems, but there is also a *skill* that comes from being adequately prepared for succeeding tasks. Skill is a horizontal strategy that is difficult to detect in the way that we identify strategies in cross section from time to time. I emphasize the skill that is used throughout life because it is the *bridge* between biological endowment and intentional behavior. It is the artful deployment of appropriate strategies, linking the organic and psychosocial. When, for example, we reflect on past life, with its mistakes, regrets, and lost opportunities, it is, in fact, a rueful review of how poor our understanding was and how unskillfully we coped with problems that should have been recognized.

Psychosocial adaptation

The term *psychosocial* refers to every element within the social and psychological field that is not strictly physical and organic.

It also means the teleological part of the life cycle, including how a person gets along and is expected to behave in the community or other social organization. But skipping over inadequate academic attempts to define what is meant by psychosocial, I believe that it is the emotional and social counterpart of physical well-being and health. Consequently, whatever it takes to be human is psychosocial in some respect.

On the other hand, psychosocial is a term to apologize for, since it grafts different disciplines and excludes others. Nature recognizes no such split between the biological and the psychosocial. You and I, for instance, are certainly biopsychosocial creatures but much more. Never will we be accounted for, or count for very much, simply by stringing prefixes together and calling it a discipline.

Psychosocial adaptation is to be lived as a unity and not as a collection of parts. It is the index of organic meaning that humanizes information of all kinds. If, for example, Thanksgiving were not celebrated until we understood fully the sociology of holidays and folk customs, the ornithology of turkeys, and the planting and harvesting of various traditional vegetables, this favorite American holiday that is an institutionalized psychosocial unit would justifiably disappear, if indeed it could be conceived at all. It would be too tedious to understand, let alone to participate in. Instead, happily, Thanksgiving is a creation or context of lived-through organic meanings that decide how we conduct ourselves on this day. When various events finally jell, lived-through participation is unified into a psychosocial event.

Adaptation is also a somewhat tedious, overworked, and redundant concept, because basically it is the name given to successfully coping with potentially damaging events. But over the longitudinal course of finding and dealing with states of progressive psychosocial disequilibrum, adaptation is the best term we have, provided that we recognize its open-ended and evanescent characteristics.

Psychosexual fulfillment

No better example of biological, social, psychological, and emotional unification can be imagined than sexuality. I need not justify the reality of a psychosexual subcycle, which has distinctive problems and strategies to cope with. Sex, sexuality, reproduction, eroticism, love, and all their derivatives constitute an awesome subcycle. Even referring to sexual "acts of participation" in a psychosocial unit sounds ludicrously pedantic. However, whether sexuality is consuming, mystifying, or mundane in its sweep and pervasiveness, it is only a subcycle, not an entire life cycle.

During adolescence and young adulthood, the preemptive presence of sexuality, from the viewpoint of both rutting and romance, encourages the belief that it encompasses everything and is everything. Sexuality during this period is literally like a religion, often with its own theology and acolytes. Nevertheless, young people could be induced to believe in Marxist determinism, if they were hungry, ill-housed, impoverished and deprived. Hunger, too, is a recurrent appetite, though not with the same mores, morals, and machinery available to sexuality.

The juices of passionate eroticism are not the life blood of sexuality. Ethology has demonstrated that even in so-called lower animals, instinct is far from blind passion to couple and reproduce. Instinct is rather well-organized, socialized behavior, constituting species-specific preparation for a number of roles, including that of parenting the young.

Psychosexuality and its fulfillment, as humans know, is consummated and conveyed in numerous biological and nonbiological contexts. Customs, morals, economics, conduct all help to conspire with hormones to decide how mankind shall perpetuate itself and provide individual humans with sexual fulfillment. Reproduction is only a small element of human psychosexuality.

The psychosexual subcycle undergoes enormous change in form, intensity, object, goal, and direction throughout the life cycle. It becomes less and less of one thing, more and more of another. The organic meaning of participation in a psychosocial unit also changes. Only the gender remains the same, with certain noteworthy exceptions. As years pass, the incandescence of sexuality yields to a no less passionate conjugation and bonding, over time, of one person with another.

The aberrations, sublimations, and directions of sexuality spread to become a comprehensive libidinal field that endows experience with a sense of reality. Sexual attraction starts with tiny buds along the urogenital tract and proliferates beyond the body to most spheres of life. Sexual pleasure is nature's bribe to perpetuate itself. Propagation is important to nature, but nature is also profligate in wasting lives.

From the viewpoint of old age, what once seemed like a compelling and undifferentiated instinctive force not to be denied is revealed to be extremely diversified as well as sterotyped. Old age sees that psychosocial forces also exert much pressure to determine specific kinds of partners. Choices at one phase of the subcycle may not even be tolerable at another. Mating and marriage may grow further apart. In our culture, at least, people seem to have better reasons for getting a divorce than to get married. In neither case is reproduction cited as a compelling reason.

In old age psychosexuality has no place for emotional bribery, guilt, blackmail, or illusion. At the end of the subcycle, reasonably compatible people find themselves bonded in intimacy and attachment. Liberation from more tempestuous signs of sexuality has its value. There is only room for unending wonderment about how we acquire, form, and use our emotional allegiances.

Racial, ethnic, cultural, and tribal et ceteras

This complex subcycle, stemming from psychosocial and psychosexual sources, contains so many factors and contingencies that variations spoil our favorite hypotheses about so-called "human nature." We glibly talk about what should happen, about "everyone," and "everywhere," seldom realizing that what seems perfectly acceptable in one section of the globe is unthinkable in another community.

I emphasize "et ceteras" and give them equal status with more familiar rubrics such as race, culture, ethnicity, and, of course, provinciality. These factors endow people with characteristics and coping styles that are so ingrained as to be correctly called second nature. Heterogeneity produces traditions, customs, rules, and traits, including values and opportunities, that cover everything from tribal roles to geographical adaptation.

Et ceteras do not need further documentation of diverse traits, customs, and characteristics that determine the expectable problems indigenous to a special group. My list of expectable problems (Chapter 2) is not, however, likely to be significantly changed, because it refers to issues that would apply anywhere. Fortunately, not being a cultural anthropologist, I can take certain liberties that specialists cannot. For example, I would have to document what seems self-evident. Among self-evident examples are those that try to prove or argue from analogy that one group within a specific society is like another for the same reasons. Generalizations are, of course, likely to be deceptive and false with respect to races and cultures just as much as forced comparisons between religions and nationalities are apt to be artificial. The uniqueness of lived-through experience, even that of a special group, will or should prevent us from forcing a hypothesis into a familiar mold. Et ceteras make things and people unique in their lived-through acts of participation. Their expectable problems will greatly differ, but certain overall fears, say, about disability, serious sickness, death, and so forth are apt to be familiar.

Therefore, whether the idea violates our sense of human community or not, it is as difficult to understand, empathize with or participate in the thinking, customs, and emotions of another group, with respect to lived-through experience, as to turn inside out. Translations always suffer from the same trouble—translation. Individual subcycles resemble each other only as all snowstorms are alike; each flake is different, and the amount of snow is only a trace of the storm itself. If we are accustomed to local weather-watching, we cannot comprehend larger concepts of climate.

Et ceteras open us to still other viewpoints. Science, philosophy, art, and other graceful disciplines elevate us beyond our localities and special provinces, exposing us to a wider sense of affiliation. But to feel universality is not the same as to understand how one person lives and another dies.

I do not and cannot wholly understand the motives of mankind, nor even the way that men and women think who live only a mile or two from where I am now. Empathy and intuition are dignified, well-intentioned words that designate our reaching for an understanding. They do not guarantee getting it.

Honesty requires that we use our system of coping with expectable problems, as determined by the racial, ethnic, and all other et ceteras that make us unique.

The system also uses us, as we use the system. Even our rebellions take on an appropriate coloration that only is a reinforcement of the system. Lived-through experiences are typical only within the singular group system of et ceteras and expectable problems. Alienation among Aleuts is likely to be as devastating and demoralizing as alienation among college students in Boston. But cultural characteristics and coping strategies are certainly much different, even if external manifestations of vulnerability resemble each other. For example, suicide is a universal instance of noncoping and vulnerability. There is scarcely a case for enlightened extinction. Nevertheless, reasons given for self-destruction, such as frustrated love, unmitigated hate, despair, as well as for alcoholism, drug addiction, and other kinds of distress, are individualized. The mortar and pestle of each society, with its et ceteras, will grind individuals down into uniquely experienced fears and problems. Their journey toward limbo covers different terrains. That which is mundane and commonplace for me may be incomprehensible to you, and the reverse is also true. Asking what makes people so disaffiliated and estranged is the wrong question. They begin that way; mothers and children do not speak the same language, and it takes considerable time before the child becomes socialized into conformity with common meanings and values. Estrangement is seldom overcome completely. It is somewhat miraculous that we communicate at all.

Ideological affiliations

Racial, ethnic, cultural, and tribal et ceteras will, most certainly, strongly determine what any of us believes and professes, quite apart from our inner estrangement. Our principles are but precipitates of earlier lived-through events, combined with peculiarities of upbringing and diversified indoctrination.

Ideology is the product of an earlier mix of many et ceteras, beyond enumeration. We are likely to be persuaded by what we already believe. Ideological affiliations go through a distinctive subcycle and leave tracks indicating where we have been and what we have gone through. Beliefs are not based on cool, detached, organized observations but are decided only by what is in our best interest to believe, according to the stage of the underlying subcycle. For example, I can readily believe, and would never consider doubting, that the earth is round and that water is H_2O. I need no proof because these facts are consistent with the world I live in. I can also entertain new notions, provided that they do not challenge or transgress my sense of reality. I can convince you of my beliefs only when I find a point of entry into your sense of reality. Otherwise, you believe correctly that I am mistaken.

Like old loves and new attachments, ideological affiliations change and remain the same, sequestered and untended, but thoroughly viable when the occasion demands.

Young rebels become more conservative, pious adolescents turn into middle-aged skeptics, romantics relinquish illusions but may be enraptured by still other visions. Traces of one kind of lived-through experience persist in some instances, but become converted into their unlived equivalents later on. Ideas are ready to change, crossing over in lived-through events.

Consider the uncounted multitudes who throughout history have died for causes not understood, forgotten, or merely fabricated as pretexts by tyrants. They died in carrying out a coping strategy picked for them in order to deal with an ideological affiliation. Prejudices, bias, stereotypes, dogmas, and a host of *-isms* denote ideologies that incline toward specific actions and away from certain problems. Great issues and momentous controversies are seldom resolved. Only ideologies change, and then usually in response to tangential forces. But as a result, new ways to cope and affiliate present themselves. The Nazis legitimized cruelty for many Germans; as a result, reasonable, often highly intelligent people changed their beliefs and practiced genocide.

Poetry yields to practicality whenever we find that life does not scan smoothly. More urgent forces produce new forms of coping with the world as it is. Conversely, however, hard-shelled materialism may mellow with time, as everything contains its plausible opposite.

We are all rooted in the lived and unlived scripts and soil of biology and ideology, conferred upon us by many subcycles merging together. When I feel constancy in my identity, I can risk revising ideologies. But if my identity is imperiled, as when facing expectable problems, then I hold onto ideology. Many psychoanalytic hours are spent with patients who cannot decide between the life they lived and the idealized life unlived. They are torn between conflicting ideologies and identities that turn out to be different versions of each other. However, if psychoanalysis works well, ideologies broaden, affiliations are more lenient, options become more ample, and self-judgment softens. By relying less on fixed ideological positions, the subcycle moves on and the fortunate individual becomes free to experiment with other coping strategies.

Personal and mental distinction

Each subcycle finds a kind of justification in the distinctions between people who are otherwise quite similar. Thus, the subcycle of chronological uniformity amid change applies to everyone, while ideological affiliations are more individualized than racial, ethnic, cultural, and tribal et ceteras.

Beyond vague predispositions, generic distinctions, however profuse, do not account for individual traits and characteristics. Yet this is the goal of anyone who works in the field of human endeavors. For example, the concept of personality types has intrigued thinkers since ancient times. The theory of humors and that of genotypes are efforts to link group traits and tendencies to the distinctive identity of the individual.

Those who work in any of the fields of human endeavor strive to find common characteristics, largely to account for other individuals, seldom for themselves. Quest for the secret of personal and mental distinctiveness and distinction is a search for significant identity above the crowd and beyond the destiny of the species. One of the paradoxical conditions of being alive is that as we search for what makes for distinctiveness, we cannot tolerate too much similarity or difference from each other.

We belong to and are represented by many more groups and subsets than we are comfortable with. There are, in fact, more personality types than zip codes (to which, by the way, typologies have more than a passing resemblance). The unspoken intent of people who look for distinctive types among mankind is to find the exact identifying marks that would locate any individual, starting with a large geographical shelf and narrowing the search down to and through the zip code to the street, house, and room in which you are now sitting.

Where is personal and mental distinction to be found? Almost everything and every force in society pushes us to conformity and conventionality. There are style makers in personology who are as arbitrary, dictatorial, ambitious, and intolerant as any other leader who imposes his will and taste on multitudes. Fashions in personal traits considered worth emulating are as evanescent as fashions in clothes, and for much the same reason. We are told how we are supposed to think, feel, judge, and be thought of, in order to belong to the "acceptable" level of society that values us. The style-fascists, as someone once called them, are found in every field, imposing their private concepts of normality and distinction. By distributing various notions of behavior and conduct that are approved and discouraged, they advocate or dismiss certain styles of coping.

It is not too cynical to realize how pervasive and life-long are our efforts to belong, fit in, change and represent one group over another. Yielding to popular pressure in order to assure mental and personal acceptability is a generic distinction in itself. Even the clothes and costumes we wear tend to identify groups with similar ideas and allegiances. The distinction is conferred by separation of one group from another not wearing the same uniform. Teams have uniforms, but then so do people who drive the same cars, wear similar hair styles, use the same expressions that represent seniority, social and financial status, advanced thinking, and so forth, endlessly.

Mental and personal distinction may seem like a curious subcycle, since it varies with such arbitrary indifference to larger questions. But it is no less strange than the quest for personal identity through shifting ideological allegiances. Perhaps because the term *personality* means just about anything, it would be accurate to use a term such as *personal style* to capture the essence of distinction over time.

Style has more permanence, at least for the individual who would be recognizable over time. It does not fluctuate or vibrate with indecision and disapproval as much as stylish ways of dressing and thinking. Style is about as close as we can get to appreciating the unique distinction between people close up. If, for example, I try to find and state generalizations about six people I know well, it would be very difficult to go beyond a few mundane generic traits. They might all have doctoral degrees, work in professions in the neighborhood of Boston, be of a certain age, and have predictable political affiliations. But very little of what I generalize about would narrow down to their distinction, each from the other. The problem, however, is not with the generalizations but with the difficulty we have in characterizing a personal style. Style consists of salient observations about how a person copes with distinctive problems within his special domain, and this is apt to evolve over time as these problems and plights present themselves.

Personal style shows itself in many, often unexpected ways. For example, there are styles in psychiatric diagnosis, implying that styles of suffering are subject to distinctive generalizations.

As a result, a psychiatric diagnosis is a form of blaming a person for having an uncomfortable style. A patient also might blame himself for suffering in the way he does. Social approval may depend on whether one's style is consistent with other values. An irascible man, for instance, is likely to be avoided, but if he is also powerful and prestigious, his offensive, rude manner may be tolerated, perhaps even admired and emulated.

Any distinction can be reversed by using a proper context of interpretation, just as an irritable but powerful man can be praised for "having high standards." Arrogance is confidence; timidity is caution; the best is worst. Redefinition cuts in both directions, especially for mental and personal distinction and style. Thus, with the development of old age, certain personal characteristics change; identity and style remain more or less intact. But the context of interpretation for old age will, almost certainly, change because of bias about advanced age and its reputed rigidities. It is said, for example, that as people grow older, their ideas become more conservative, less tolerant and lenient. They may be suspicious of novelty and angry about deviation from routine. Other older people seemingly become more judicious and forbearing.

Now, there is nothing about aging that confers wisdom. Old people do not automatically become smarter, in the way that most adolescents have acne. Nevertheless, it is common for older people to be more subdued, probably related to physical limitations. Problems that were once very distressing lose their urgency. I favor the hypothesis that there is a subcycle for personal style and mental distinction. Changes are the result of transformations in other subcycles, but style is apt to retain its own typical configuration, coupled, of course, to the erosions of time. Still unsettled and unsettling is the awareness that various subcycles are returning to the completion of separate orbits, in preparation.

Politico-economic deployment

I do not propose that political or economic problems constitute a separate life subcycle. However, their resolution is essential at every phase for harmonious well-being and personal safety. Just as physical well-being and health are subcycles, so too are economic and political security. Integrity of the life cycle depends on financial concerns and political struggles, though not in the customary sense. If anyone doubts this statement, ask any older person or minority citizen about who is vulnerable on money matters, who is powerless in complicated society, who is impaired in confronting pressing problems of security, safety, housing, purchasing power.

Politico-economic deployment is not just a matter of how one votes or budgets money. As a subcycle it refers to recognizing and using power intelligently. It also means the ability to govern well, without being mastered or becoming indentured. Everyone, to some extent, has options pertaining to the conditions of survival. Governing oneself is a primary consideration in every area of life. This is a significant factor at any age and stage. For a child, financial resources are indirect but very real. Flexible deployment of power is more direct, becoming more localized later on, and is also very real. Politico-economic deployment means, therefore, how one distributes the power that ensures a measure of freedom, while yielding a required amount of control to the group. This is political power in its basic sense.

There is no institution that is free of political and economic strife. Distribution of power in its various forms typifies group pressures. Moreover, lofty and idealistic aims are still held together by money. Prestige, acclaim, patronage, possessions are only a few of the positions of power that most people bow down to. When considered as a subcycle, politico-economic deployment projects power longitudinally, thereby maintaining control. Presumably, power protects freedom, but it is usually the freedom of individuals possessing that power. Enlightened self-interest is about the best we can hope for, judging from the past and anticipating the new century. We also must trust, however warily, that those in power will permit us to exercise residual freedom for what matters most to us. Beyond this, it is unlikely that the good will drive out the bad in a reversal of Gresham's Law.

Fear of old age comes from many sources, including difficulties in the far end of the politico-economic subcycle. Along with reduced physical stamina, older people usually have diminished financial power as well as limited prestige, political strength, and freedom. As a result, choice, control, and sustained identity are threatened.

Diminution in politico-economic power is due to personal devaluation. The thought that we can retire from work and get more satisfaction elsewhere is a politico-economic misconception, although quality of life may improve. The real problem is how to maintain status and prestige, along with security and personal distinction. Better use and distribution of power for the aged depend on strategies that protect autonomy and minimize submission. Of course, total freedom to choose among very many options is an illusion, but by using such power as remains, the aged can arrange a mutual exchange. The pragmatism inherent in being aged is clearly shown by increasing political awareness that must be heeded by elected officials.

Thanatologic realization

The gathering shadows of old age make it imperative to retain power to act on one's own behalf. The meaning of thanatologic realization is based on disclosure of the reality of death itself. This does not come instantaneously. Realization makes real gradually by a growing appreciation that death brings every other subcycle to its natural conclusion.

Having lived through and participated in every subcycle, it is a measure of living well that we find a suitable counterpart in appropriate death. The life cycles are thereby consummated, and a good death becomes their ultimate credential.

At the end of the journey toward limbo, shadow and substance become indistinct. Although alienation and annihilation are there to adumbrate the negative side of whatever we do or fail to do at any period, the wish to leave a mark is not the same as wanting to postpone death indefinitely.

Eternal life is a promise as suitable for hell as heaven. Death and dying can be wholly acceptable. Not only will we then be beyond disease, including cancer, but we shall have triumphed over suffering and death. Consequently, the end of every subcycle is to realize that death is and can be an existential punctuation for every statement.

Thanatologic realization is a genuine subcycle for many reasons. It signifies how subcycles are woven together, spun out over years, and now snipped away, just as the Fates intended all along. I am sure that there are many more than ten subcycles. The ten-speed life cycle does not take us very far, only far enough to reaffirm our fallibility and limitations. That we are transient cannot be disputed. It even has an aesthetic appeal. At times, admittedly, faced with seemingly amorphous misfortune, the Fates are like three weary women toiling in a mythological sweatshop somewhere. They are forever gathering threads and cloth, sewing them together, then ripping them apart. It seems quite futile.

Let us remember that these subcycles and indeed the life cycle as a whole are very crude images. It is obvious that the purpose of subcycles is to provide a sense of harmony over time in our efforts to cope with a sequence of expectable problems. Self-identity exerts selective emphasis over which subcycle seems more important. Consequently, when the realization of death becomes uppermost, we will understand, in retrospect, how we have shaped the outcome according to our personal meanings and intentions. The realization of death transcends the fading memories of those who survive us. Its surplus, highly personal significance can make us content with oblivion.

CHAPTER 7

THE SURVIVAL
OF THE DODO

It should be clear by now that there is no grand, encompassing life cycle that arches over us like a rainbow in the sky. The trajectory of expectable changes during anyone's life span cannot be predicted with regularity. There are just too many idiosyncrasies, unanticipated events, blips, peaks, and valleys.

Life cycles and subcycles are mainly ways to think about basic strategies that map the contours of how we ordinarily deal with typical tasks and problems. The noiseless unfolding of events, year after year, gathers direction from whatever goes before. When these events seem orderly, their distribution is called development and maturation. In truth, however, inheritance is only part of the plan. There are imprints, as well as capricious occasions and accidents that shift development into different channels. And we cannot ignore the conflicts, contentions, and compromises that enter into reasons for survival.

An extraterrestrial observer, or what is more plausible, an earthly inhabitant seeking a longer perspective, must arrive at a rather simple conclusion, considering the complexity. The conclusion is that man requires a great deal of ingenuity and fortitude to survive his own mistakes, violence, and fallibility.

Because of an endless assortment of perplexing tasks, we must also infer that the purpose of such abundant activity is to cope well enough and nurture morale high enough to endure disappointment and despair.

Coping well enough is therefore a matter of developing morale strong enough. Assuming that you are faced with a serious problem, what could be done that will be worthy of you at your best? Favorite strategies are personal benchmarks distinctive enough to typify your style over time. As a rule, only good friends are familiar enough with our style to recognize the strategies embedded in what we say and do. But even good friends may not be objective enough to understand the situations that evoke characteristic strategies. For example, when a man's style is to wait for serious problems and choices to be decided for him, friends may simply think that he is prudent and does not want to make mistakes. This is true, but in addition the passive strategy exempts him from blame and deprives him of the satisfaction of having risked and then found a significant reward. Friends may not see how deviously he seeks advice and allows them to propose a course of action.

Coping strategies are unique and stereotyped, a melange of custom and convenience, opportunity and obligation. As noted earlier (Chapter 3), even the fifteen rather simple strategies seldom appear in pure form. Rather, they come together in clusters, clump, fractionate, and then rearrange themselves in novel patterns. But their overriding purpose is the same: to pursue a solution that is within the scope of being at one's best, while restoring a measure of equilibrium.

The best assessment of how worthwhile our values have been occurs at that distant point where subcycles coincide and subside in old age. If the values sought throughout life are truly substantial, not just bitter reminders of irreversible mistakes, then the larger strategies we adopted were worthwhile. They acquire a patina of authenticity, indicating that for the most part morale has been sustained.

Coping in itself is not a significant goal. But good coping enables us to link primary motivations with ultimate resolutions of problems getting in the way. Good copers use a more extensive array of *intermediate* strategies than those who perforce are limited to a very few that may not be flexible enough to survive. Here is a list of intermediate strategies, but I ask my readers to readers to remember that self-instruction demands that they observe what works best for them. In addition, it is useful to develop a good-natured skepticism about any strong recommendations, lest we fall into the passive goal of having decisions made for us and lose genuine freedom to choose.

INTERMEDIATE STRATEGIES

1. Set a goal.
   Imagine an aim, purpose, or goal that lines up with a more distant objective; but because coping is not a mechanism or an exercise in engineering, be prepared to adopt a secondary goal. Self-instruction is to develop skill in many potential strategies.
2. Monitor results.
   Check the effectiveness of intermediate strategies because revision may be necessary.
3. Confront, correct, redefine.
   By examining what one does, one can at times transform problems into a more positive set of issues that are coped with more readily.
4. Keep composure.
   Composure means even-tempered caution, not artificial serenity and calm under all circumstances.
5. Preserve primary morale.
   Coping well is based on believing, first of all, that coping well enough is possible. Then, does this way of behaving represent you at your best? Being at one's best is never absolute nor is it always possible. It is something to strive for, although it is not the ideal.

Secondary morale is using the approval of others who seemingly are with you for mutual purposes.

6. Do what is practical and feasible.

Trust not to luck. Do not depend on a *deus ex machina*, guardian angel, or emulate Mr. Micawber waiting for something to turn up. Instead, when faced with prospective failure, ask, "What can be done now? What are my options?" Having failed, ask what you have learned in order to prevent future failure.

7. Cultivate confidence.

Confidence does not breed arrogance nor does resignation mean acceptance of tragedy. Aptitude is no guarantee that all will be well. Confidence in coping is a prerequisite for coping well; fatalism is defeat posing as a philosophy.

8. Use collaboration.

Self-reliance is an absolute, but to feel utterly independent is self-deception absolute. Good copers usually use others whose skills, knowledge, and intentions deserve trust and respect.

9. Develop other strategies.

Regardless of how well we cope, backup plans are always necessary, as long as a problem remains. These alternatives should be varied enough to contend with unexpected circumstances. Resourceful simply means to have more resources. Incessant worry is usually futile, since it frets about hidden dangers without finding practical steps that supplement and strengthen strategies already in use.

10. There are no absolutes.

Solutions are never permanent, nor are good copers always adept at solving problems. Respect for limitations and trust in being able to survive helps confront fallibility. But tragedy happens, anyway; seldom do we have much to do about it, except to revise and redefine our skill and style.

These intermediate strategies may be difficult to practice and put into action, but each can be used selectively until they fuse into a formidable set of attitudes that promote problem-solving. Good copers do not strive for the unattainable, which only mocks their efforts, like Hobson's choice without a horse for hire.

I have frequently alluded to *being at one's best*. This is no visionary goal, suitable only for idealists or saints who are not called on to do anything and never have to compromise. It is a product of cultivating versatility, openmindedness, skepticism, and resiliency, and still being able to imagine whether being at one's best is really feasible. Acceptance of fallibility does not demand self-condemnation for not being or reaching perfection. He who tries to walk on water usually finds that he gets his feet wet and should wonder why he tried it in the first place.

WHAT DID THE DODO IN?

Once upon a time there was the dodo, a flightless, inedible bird inhabiting a remote island in the Indian Ocean called Mauritius. Soon after man settled the island, bringing in other rapacious animals, the dodo became extinct. Apparently, it did not or could not escape. Now it lives on only in legend, "dead as a dodo."

There was no obvious reason for destroying these harmless birds, except that they were harmless and vulnerable. Presumably, other animals on the island survived by being secretive, resourceful, or powerful enough to cope successfully. The dodo was none of these.

I am, to be sure, not a naturalist, but I am curious about this legendary bird. What led to its failure to cope better? What did the dodo do that did it in? We do not know if the dodo tried any strategies except the ones that failed. If we had been dodos, could we have learned anything to help prevent failure and to reduce vulnerability?

Maybe before the dodo was completely exterminated, it expected man to change his ways by becoming more merciful or less violent, or even to be distracted by other things to do. If the dodo did so, then it adopted ruinous behavior and encouraged its own destruction.

Lewis Carroll also wondered about the poor dodo and inadvertently, I believe, suggested what troubled the creature. Carroll's dodo either devised or proposed the famous Caucus Race, for no particular reason. By design, it seemed, the race was haphazard; it had no rules and could not be won by the swift, strong, smart, stealthy, skillful, or even the lucky. The race began and ended abruptly. The course went this way and that, turning back on itself, finishing nowhere in particular. Who won? Who lost? After a great deal of thought, the dodo proposed, "Everybody has won, and all must have prizes!"

This decision, elevated to the status of a principle, clearly goes against our beliefs in competition, survival of the fittest, and the virtue in being a victor. If we do not believe that winning is everything, what is the purpose of competition? Losing does not have much to recommend it.

As befits such a race, the dodo's prizes that everybody deserved were pretty meager. In my opinion, however, the dodo was trying to make a point. No one lost—whatever that meant—but by participating in a race without rules over a chaotic course, a case could be made for awarding prizes to everyone. ("I again saw under the sun that the race is not to the swift, and the battle is not to the warriors, and neither is bread to the wise, nor wealth to the discerning, nor favor to men of ability; for time and chance overtake them all."—*Ecclesiastes*, 9:11).

Nevertheless, the very notion that no one can be a loser seems heretical nonsense. No wonder then that the dodo is extinct. It makes much more sense to advise: cope as if your life depended on it, because it does. The dodo might still be alive, had this advice been given and heeded.

The principle of competition, which means winning and losing, success and failure, has more advocates than those who actually practice the Golden Rule, which, if conscientiously followed, might revolutionize mankind. The Golden Rule, however, is not the Dodo's Rule, because, if everybody won, deserving or not, who would have the benefits and acclaim that the world confers?

Even a game must have problems to cope with, but to do so requires at least rudimentary knowledge of the rules and objectives, in addition to skill.

But imagine that the Dodo's Rule could be applied, here and there. The stronger would take care of the weaker, the wise look after the foolish, the rich provide for the poor. Giving prizes to all might even help the inept losers. Survival of the sickest would not merely be a product of philanthropy but the reigning philosophy and ethical directive.

Before deciding about these opposing doctrines of survival, let us also imagine what might occur were life in fact a Caucus Race. There would be unspecified rules, incomprehensible aims, arbitrary directions, chaotic guidelines, unmethodical orders, and abrupt endings. Moreover, to proclaim everybody a winner would be meaningless, because the prizes were trivial. Consequently, because no rules applied, nothing would make any difference, nor should we care very much. Random events hardly constitute problems worth coping with.

Come to think about it, isn't this somewhat like what most of us already contend with? Our future fate is certainly very obscure, the plan of life is unpredictable, what we do often lacks specific purpose, and our final things are quite elusive, if indeed we know what they are.

The life cycle, ten-speed or not, is like a Caucus Race. Rules mean little, directives are either vague or inapplicable, expedients pose as principles, and consensus means only that we agree on what is convenient and comfortable.

I could go on with seemingly paradoxical outcomes of the Dodo's Rule: the good die young, evil triumphs, virtue has its painful rewards, and blessings come unnecessarily well disguised. Like Alice, we are lucky to get our own thimble back. However, according to the philosophy of the Winner, everybody else is a loser and all must forfeit.

Let us now assume that the dodo soberly invented the Caucus Race in order to symbolize or put into metaphorical reality its ineptitude in coping. The race would have its origin in a real event, often lost to memory. Mythology is full of such inventions.

Like an obsessional ritual or compulsive practice, the game would undo a painful event, such as the destruction of the dodo. The race memorializes a lost cause, not just ineffective coping. My guess is that the lost cause is futile, meaningless, random activity to no purpose whatsoever. If no rules exist or are too obscure to fathom, there is nothing to lose or gain. Coping would be meaningless. The dodo merely plays out its historical tragedy over and over, conveying the message that dodo-kind must yield to the inevitability of destruction and nothing can be done about it. The dodo might have had the fate of slaves on Mauritius in mind. Around the time of the dodo's demise, the slaves won a kind of symbolic freedom by becoming "indentured workers." Their status was redefined, a strategy we are already familiar with. Whether this conferred a genuine prize is doubtful, but at least they survived.

The Dodo's doctrine might have appealed to a distant cousin named Candide, who believed that everything and everyone fitted into a pattern. He held that things happen for a purpose, however inscrutable, and therefore in the sense that they happen, they happen for the best, regardless of suffering and pain entailed.

Candide's philosophy has several implications. It may be a modest version of the idea that those who survive are best equipped to survive, cope best of all, and therefore deserve to survive while others perish. A second implication is that those who win are undoubtedly the rulers, and those who do not are subjects. Although Candide concluded that tending one's own garden was advisable (CS 5 & 8), countless rulers and kings never made the history books. Their causes were obscure at best. But they killed each other just the same and massacred multitudes who, I fear, thought that what they did was meritorious. Candide missed the point: when rulers kill other rulers and cause their subjects to be killed, it is because man exploits his fellow man in order to get what he wants. I leave it to my readers to identify the coping strategies involved.

Job had a similar problem about trying to understand the nature of evil. In my opinion, the closest we have come to understanding the various ways in which evil is packaged is to change its name.

Calling a slave an "indentured worker" may help someone, but probably only a conscience-stricken master who prefers to be called an employer with a comprehensive work schedule. Because we do not know which rules apply to specific situations, it is difficult to tell whether absolute standards exist or just that our methods of judgment are weak. Some coping strategies are definitely better than others. The intermediate strategies clearly are better suited for confrontation, clarification, and appropriate action based on what is practical, feasible, and likely to ensure significant survival. As another endangered species, we can learn from the dodo's fate. It is very cold comfort to imagine a future in which progress will be unmistakable, since our methods for correcting evils are not only rudimentary but largely ignored.

COPING WITH COEXISTENCE

After all, I suppose that our life cycles are like heedless, headlong, random, and meaningless Caucus Races in which very few people do very well. There are prizes and penalties for everybody, and they are distributed and awarded in obscure ways, not always based on merit. What are the alternatives?

One alternative that the dodo might have considered is to work out an agreement with predators so that we can survive. Obviously, the only ones likely to be convinced are those from whom we expect no harm. Another alternative is to get away from the winner-take-all philosophy, cultivate self-identity, cope with coexistence, and avoid exterminating each other. Since we are not aware of absolute truths or standards that everyone understands and acts on, our obligation is coping as well as possible with problems that can be identified.

Is mutual survival through coping with coexistence too much or too little to strive for? It has the advantage of clarity in that we will understand the purpose of coexistence, which is *maintenance of mutual morale*, without the dubious benefit of selective decimation through combat. Everybody's prize would be a better quality and quantity of life.

Mutuality is the antithesis of sublimated combat. It does not require killing or even humiliating an opponent. Domination is superfluous. Then who shall lead us? A freely chosen leader of limited strength but infinite wisdom is a naive prospect. In the animal kingdom, leaders become too old, overconfident, too entrenched, and then are easily displaced. Ultimately, to win is to lose. But need the fact of losing invite destruction, disaster, and death? Can the subcycles be permitted to wind down and quietly consummate themselves on the altar of an appropriate death in which we all participate? The consummation of every coping strategy and the culmination of reduced vulnerability are freedom with coexistence, free from coercion and competition.

Is man capable of this goal? True to the disguises that evil so jauntily wears, at the end of this century monarchs have been supplanted by authoritarians who glibly talk about freedom and open institutions. We choke on platitudes.

The dodo is dead. So is Candide, and Job has many descendants no more fortunate or wiser than he. Meanwhile, I endorse such viewpoints as coping with coexistence, knowing that this motto is not more substantial than any other pleasant aroma from the kitchen of thought. We sniff, and then it blows away.

Nevertheless, the quest for morale cannot be disregarded, because it has eminent practical applications. We simply cannot in our transience be totally obliterated by other life cycles bearing down on us. Coexistence is difficult, but to cope well demands close adherence to the ideal of better morale, being at or near one's best under a wide range of circumstances, with diverse problems.

Cultivation of better morale requires endless, interminable self-exploration, using every strategy that can be mustered, nourished, and put into practice. Otherwise, we capitulate to the brutes, and like the harmless, vulnerable dodo, play out a pointless game.

On this island, not even despair can be counted on. Cynics must yield to their own sense of futility, because our task is to find steps leading to the values worth pursuing. One of these steps is the distinction between *competition* and *coexistence*. Competition threatens the survival of the sickest, while coexistence means that in a close race most of us would not do very well.

Perhaps the distinction is analogous to the difference between irony and sarcasm, which are two superficially similar ways of dissembling. Irony means coexistence with another person whom we treat with good-natured mockery, while tolerating a faulty situation. Sarcasm is much meaner, aiming to destroy while disguised as irony. It is hostile and intended to tear someone apart. I prefer irony, hands down. Sarcasm does not permit us even to retaliate, an inexcusable state in which all bleeding is internal. Very insecure people are threatened by irony because they do not understand it and feel they are being affronted and attacked. For them, coexistence is out of the question. In their eyes freedom is liberty to exploit those too weak to defend themselves. As a result, because they feel among the weakest, insecurity breeds more coercion. Insecurity is another synonym for poor morale and, of course, inability to use good coping strategies.

Competition is no more valid a law of nature than the freedom to kill because we are threatened and have no other strategies to use. An animal's so-called drive to kill is rather selective, as I understand it, and is hardly comparable to man's drive to dominate, exploit, exterminate. Coexistence can become a custom as deeply honored and established as coercion. I believe there are prizes enough to go around, just as amply as penalties.

A favorable existentialist chant is being here-and-now. We dwell in an amorphous future and gather guidelines from a skewed past; thus we construct the present. The "gift of life" is not a present but the *presence* of an unblinkable fact that we are that life. There is no other moment but *now*, except that what is coped with now is a preparation for problems still to come. To do so effectively, we negotiate with coexistence.

A more somber, yet trenchant synonym for the collective subcycles is called the journey toward limbo. It is neither a fate nor a consolation, but it does require a certain capacity to recollect past problems and reevaluate the course of events. This is best done from the standpoint of old age, provided we are honest and candid enough to see that despite good intentions our best efforts do not invariably succeed.

Limbo is an abode of souls who are eligible for neither heaven nor hell. Through no grievous fault of their own, there they remain, never to be reprieved. I am not, of course, describing the theological meaning of limbo but that of a more humanistic world between heaven and hell and therefore neutral. It is a concept completely compatible with the neutrality of the here-and-now and the uncertainty of the future. In this abode we cope and fail to cope well enough. We try to instruct ourselves and participate in self-exploration, in order to be better prepared for ensuing problems and dilemmas. This abode, which is *now*, is located between existence and extinction. With good morale, we can repudiate annihilation, just as we tolerate other kinds of vulnerability.

Limbo, in the secular sense, is a moment of confinement, of destiny perhaps, in which we face the restrictions of mortality. Although we are confined within a limited range of barbed-wire freedom, we are courageous and compassionate enough at times to acknowledge the absolute truth of transience and oblivion. This is our common allotment and thus the grounds for coexistence. In this century the specter of concentration camps and of incurable disease prepares us for the likelihood of nuclear incineration. Coexistence may not be possible until we recognize that these specters should rightfully haunt everyone. Everybody loses, and all shall pay penalties! Like the dodo, we have no place to hide or to flee from predators. We cannot trust in a faith that promises only an ultimate retribution or an equally remote reward. The message is too obscure. Furthermore, coexistence also means that penalties and punishment for others are not prizes for us.

DOES OLD AGE MAKE SENSE?

Old age marks the culmination, if not the consummation, of existence. It is what certifies our presence, just prior to extinction. While many old people would find the term *culmination* rather ironic, considering their depletion and decrepitude, being old is neither heaven nor hell but a mirror of limbo. Contrary to its theological meaning, my concept of a secular limbo is largely populated by old people puzzling endlessly about how they managed to live so long and for what purpose.

I have already deplored society's condescending and sometimes compassionate attitude toward even the more vigorous aged. The patronizing phrase "aging gracefully" means only that an older person makes very little noise and carries middle-age values into later years. Then, allowing for good health and enough solvency to withstand poverty, vigorous old age will be expected to combine subcycles harmoniously, so that a quiet, not too distressing exitus will be assured. At the other extreme, however, decrepit old age surely fuses invalidism, incompetence, and insolvency. Most oldsters are in between and know it.

Unless positive values justify the manifold vulnerabilities of old age, those who are advanced in years are no better off than a doddering dodo. If significant values are beyond our reach or irrelevant, then we live beyond reason, where rationality no longer applies. Coping with expectable problems is a fitting purpose at any age, but problems differ; that is the meaning of the life cycles. Only if vulnerability is kept in check, commensurate with problems coped with and consonant with unique values, will old age make sense. As a mirror of limbo, old age will reflect and assess activities that have brought that person to a penultimate point when illusions of immunity can no longer be indulged.

OMEGA VALUES AND VULNERABILITY

I am fond of the Greek letter omega, as others are who want to lend a sense of finality and importance to statements about ultimate points. But omega does not just signify finality, end, termination. Rather, I use it as a sign that conveys the completeness and closure of life, as subcycles meet and then subside.

If old age is to make sense, however, hope must prevail. Hope means that special values, unique to the aged, are there to be pursued and fulfilled. These values will differ from middle-age values carried over to old age and will have a positive significance for those hopeful and vigorous enough.

Because we have a hypocritical attitude toward aging, the values usually deferred to old age are either inspirational pap or simply the upside-down version of what might happen if an expectable problem were resolved. For example, it is pap to tell someone who is out of a job that now he can enjoy the fruits of leisure time, without knowing whether he has financial resources, social supports, housing, and so on. An upside-down version of unemployment in the aged is to propose a solution that solves nothing. Thus, if an older person is no longer employable at a respectable job, he may be urged to volunteer his services for a variety of inconsequential tasks. I do not minimize such tasks as baby-sitting, pushing wheelchairs in hospitals, and delivering messages from one office to another. But these are hardly fulfilling, and they do not preserve or enhance self-esteem and responsibility.

Whether any value is simply the reverse of a problem one wishes were not there is a theoretical question irrelevant at this point. I will offer ten suggestions that can be called omega values; namely, criteria for successful acts in old age. These should be used in conjunction with the intermediate strategies described at the start of this chapter.

Exemption from the work ethic

Exemption from the duty to work is far different from inability to find and do work that is satisfying. The work ethic has been bred strong, so that uselessness and unemployment go together, almost indistinguishably. Patronizing reassurances about deserving a rest, not needing to prove oneself, and so on, make it no easier to feel obsolete. Existence is difficult to justify when there are no socially sanctioned jobs to do. Nevertheless, it makes better coping sense for the older person to say, "I have earned the right to have another opportunity," than to brood over what has gone, including the dubious glories of the past.

Exemption from the work ethic calls upon everything else that has been developed during working years besides the skills related to earning a living. Self-esteem, which we carry forward in every subcycle, is their common quality. In old age the lived and unlived come together, since to some extent neither exists in quite the same way. The difference between them is lessened because exemption from the work ethic as an occupational directive is replaced by efforts to bolster morale. We become our own template.

Freedom for individuality

Let us never forget that everybody is forgettable, and that even the famous will dwindle within a generation or two. When viewed against the ideal, we are all anonymous, uncelebrated, pretty shabby specimens. There is very little that encourages much confidence in the importance of individuality. Indeed, individuality may merely exaggerate minor differences between one person and another.

Omega values insist that even meager prizes are worthwhile and available to all. Otherwise, except for very few, the rest of us would be losers in a race we did not understand in the first place. Authentic individuality cannot exist without feeling a right to choose a course of action and a right to coexist with others, without exploiting and being exploited. I know no better definition of freedom. This kind of freedom is not that of narcissistic entitlement. While authentic individuality needs nurturance, narcissism needs a constant fix. Entitlement is like self-pity, a somewhat argumentative demand for ego juices that other people seem to withhold.

In younger years the search for authentic individuality and the freedom to use it are cast in rebellious terms. Later on it becomes self-evident that freedom does not require the test of rebellion. Even if no one else cares, authentic individuality thrives on choosing to live within self-chosen conformity, which may be very inconspicuous and unobtrusive. It is not, however, synonymous with comfortable conventionality. The aged, for example, learn to distinguish between what is expected of them and what they really want and need. Even though the scope of choice and control is narrowed, this may not matter.

Undistracted self-instruction

Self-instruction, along with self-exploration, has been a prerequisite of good coping throughout this journey, now immersed in imminent but vigorous old age. What we endure we cope with, and survive. What we survive is a source of self-instruction. How well we self-instruct is reflected in how effectively we cope. If we cope well enough, then among other things we self-instruct and seek tolerance for ambiguity, relief of anxiety, abstention from existential envy, and the power to participate in a Caucus Race that makes very little sense.

Short-term goals and long-term motivation

The aged have time for only short-term goals but need the energy and motivation sufficient for limitless aspiration. Of course, roaring ambition subsides soon enough, long before old age quiets the tempest. Envy of the next generation cannot lead to renewed competition; that is inconsistent with omega values for which we have self-instructed. Unlimited motivation must learn to deal with foreshortened life expectancy, but there is no failure in leaving work incomplete at life's end. Warm incentives need not be reduced to cold ashes on the hearth of time. For those who are afraid of the dark, a reminder that night is falling hastens resignation. But a time for reflection is time well spent and not at all fatalistic. Old age can be a time for deliberation, not hurry, about selecting a long series of short-term goals. We are, for example, better able to appreciate what we do and might have done, thus monitoring how the unlived life still weaves itself into actuality.

While long-range resolution of eternal problems is unlikely to capture much incentive, short-term goals offer the satisfaction of knowing the approximate outcome and even provide an opportunity for rehearsing other conclusions. An elderly philosopher, hospitalized with incurable illness and unlikely to return home, told me that he hadn't any time for eternal problems; they had already taken up too much energy, more than necessary. I inferred that he meant something fairly wise by this cryptic remark. Maybe he meant that eternal problems are not problems at all but rather guidelines by which we steer a course. Having almost completed his voyage, the guidelines could now be dispensed with. The trip was over. I drew another conclusion, however: omega values are worthwhile only if they help us to participate in a compatible closure, without foreclosure on further fulfillment in short-range choices.

Uncertainty and solitude

On first glance, there is nothing very appealing or valuable about uncertainty and solitude, since we cannot be sure about ambiguity or care very much about ambivalence. To be alone with the vaguely perceived and poorly understood is hardly worthwhile. Among the platitudes pointed at the elderly, one of the favorites is that something must be done about the loneliness, solitude, uncertainty, and anxiety of old age, as if younger people had no such problems and the aged were excessively vulnerable. The opposite may be true, so far as uncertainty and solitude are concerned.

To fear solitude is to fear alienation and extinction. Many older people are taught such fears and fret about their isolation and loneliness. Childish insistence on the constant company of others leads to petulance and dogmatism, not to greater appreciation of the younger generation. Many tasks and goals require solitude, and uncertainty may spur the quest for short-term explorations. To be uncertain is still to know a great deal, just as fearing the unknown means to fear what we already know.

What most people mean by fear of the unknown, and for that matter fear of uncertainty and solitude, is the already known fact that tomorrow, or soon thereafter, the veil of uncertainty may be stripped away abruptly to reveal death itself, with its ultimate solitude. Old age finds dread of death and its denial equally difficult to maintain. But old age may forgo the *opportunity* to confront uncertainty and solitude. It is an opportunity in the short range to preserve limitless appetite for foreknowledge. In old age solitude finds that the foggy mirror of time is clear enough to recognize our own reflection starting back at us. This uplifting thought cannot be realized if we renounce uncertainty for false dogmatism about unlimited survival or if we enclose ourselves in a capsule, clustering with others.

Uncertainty and solitude can be strategic values, therefore, especially when faced with the expectable problem of loss and grief. Without adequate preparation for solitude, death and deprivation of those who meant most—those who provided a sense of reality, those who sustained our illusions—lead to demoralization. Under such circumstances survival makes hardly any sense. But with adequate capacity to tolerate uncertainty and solitude, being bereft will relinquish its place to a quiet resignation, a very good coping strategy (CS 8, with an assist from CS 7). At the very least, comfortable solitude and tolerable uncertainty remind us that a life without bereavement is hardly worth examining.

Passionate sublimation

Among omega values that counsel resignation, solitude, and undistracted self-instruction, it may seem paradoxical now to invoke passion, however qualified and presumably diluted. But passion and strong emotion are always the counterpoint to living and give thoughtfulness its thrust. That passions cool or are slow to arouse is a fact of aging that is obvious and yet hidden. Not only does this refer to manifest passions of love but to impassioned beliefs and enthusiasms, to spirited fantasies and creative improvisations. Even lust and hate are not spared as the life cycles wend themselves to a conclusion. Nevertheless, despite progressive muting and modulation of driving passions, deep attachments persist, imparting an emotional loyalty that resists the intrusions of time. The antitheses of love and hate, joy and sorrow, devotion and disdain still retain an original spirit, if not vivacity. They do not totally dwindle into pale and preoccupied neutrality.

I believe that the apathy decried in old age is probably a general indifference based on narrow interests and provincialism found in earlier life. This is, however, quite different from emotional withdrawal and self-preoccupation that occur in the very sick of any age. Sickness is no good and does nothing for anyone at any time. Those who believe in the redemptive value of suffering are most likely to find it in someone else's suffering and sickness, not their own.

It is quite natural, for example, that in the subcycle of psychosexuality, both libidinal and personal interests diminish. There are some who unnecesarily seek to assure the aged that lively sexual activity is retained until long after social security checks come in. However, for those in whom the tides of sexual passion subside, it is important to know that there is no connection between sexual activity, mental health, and a strong sense of identity and enthusiasm. Continence at any age is not harmful, just difficult. In old age libidinal interests tend to be dispersed and therefore attenuated. Were it not for the persistence of middle-age values, many older people would admit that attenuation of sexual interest is a distinct relief, although under some circumstances also regretted.

In old age psychosexuality is reduced in both urgency and viscerality. Nevertheless, deep bonding exists, less frenzied and tempestuous, less subject to oscillation, but sturdier than ever and not as prone to painful distraction.

Sublimation is real enough, just hard to define, like so many other important concepts. It differs from mere interference and inhibition of appetite and aim and from shifting of appetite and attraction to another object, more accessible. Sublimation, perhaps at every age, means to replace short-term impassioned coupling with longer-lasting bonds to a wider range of people and causes, accompanied, of course, by different activities that represent consummation. In old age an omega value in sublimation of passions is therefore likely to infuse other interests with renewed vigor, yet with restraint. I cannot wholly believe that the material for sublimation and passion is based entirely on psychosexuality, for this is but one subcycle. Other subcycles have their own impelling energy that can be deployed and shared as the course of life winds down.

Forgiving nature and tolerating mortification

This is a curious value, even for omega. It is strange, but it contributes in positive ways to the completion of life, and therefore is a positive value.

What has nature done that requires forgiveness? We can of course find ample reason to blame nature; there is nothing more tangible to blame for the injustice that is indigenous to this earth. Certainly, aside from the endless rows of victims and refugees that constitute this century, a sight that overpopulation only magnifies, the plight of only one advanced cancer patient awaiting the release of death hardly seems momentous. It would help to have something to curse and throw a stone at. The future is a most egregious illusion, except that it will happen, in one form or another. Deprivation and despair are almost like the rule of nature. Old age, of course, is not spared. Pain is never bearable, and equanimity is asking too much. Ultimately, we are usually forced to compromise with the enemy. Most of these problems are expectable (Chapter 2). They encourage yet mock our efforts to cope with them.

"Why me?" is not a question but an absurdity. Asking why is merely a plea that expects no answer. There is much to blame nature for, not the least of which is its tendency to mortify aged people seemingly as a penalty for having lived a long time. In the best of worlds, of course—which this is not—as age develops and subcycles wind down, trust and tolerance would replace angst and vulnerability. Dying then might have less pain, and death hold no fears. Death might be welcomed, like sleep for the weary and food for the hungry. Surely, there is nothing intrinsically morbid about that goal.

Mortification consists of mortality and demoralization. These afflictions represent futility of body and spirit that enfeebles when strength is most needed. How can the demoralized rise above misfortune like the Stoics of ancient times? In this sense, the best assurance of being able to cope with adversity is belief that one *can* cope, and the surest sign of despair is to be certain that one cannot. Although we are cast into the world without much apparent reason, the purpose of coping is obviously to avoid being victimized. Nature or even fate is a good target for much evil, but they are meaningless targets, and thus forgiveness is irrelevant. Forgiving nature for our fate means coming to terms with our luck, because we are either mortified by fortune or blessed by it. Blaming nature is itself a coping device (CS 13) that turns uncertainty into an evil, vengeful spirit. Forgiveness may be an antidote, but acceptance is much more effective, since we have very little opportunity to retaliate against nature or its equivalent, fate. Because, after all, nature, fate, destiny, *moira* is our construct; it is not more or less hostile and niggardly than we declare it to be. When life cycles come to a close, the urge to retaliate against any enemy relents. The wisdom of old age is based on the notion that although we can fail, falter, injure ourselves most gravely, nature is not at fault for failing to warn us. Nature promises us nothing but the fact of existence. This may not be very much, but it is not a fitting target for blame and shame.

The existential dilemma facing just about everyone is how to become reconciled to a brute fact that natural processes feel nothing and are basically indifferent, unlike what we expect our parents to feel and be. Maturity recognizes, however, that indifference is not iniquity; only man is cruel, seemingly enjoying dispensing arbitrary power and pain.

Vicarious participation

If the aged are excluded from participating in the truly important activities of life, vicarious participation simply means that they can look on, for whatever benefit that confers. But this is no great symbol of generosity and therefore not a positive value at all. Many important activities of life are not worth observing, let alone participating in. The aged would be better advised not to push forward for a good seat.

Vicarious participation has a more sanguine meaning, akin to using what trustworthy people do as a source of secondary morale; that is, feeling better about oneself through the significant activities of others. For example, very few spectators could match the performance of skilled actors, artists, musicians, and athletes. Yet under suitable circumstances onlookers gain something positive from being in the audience or on the sidelines. We can enjoy without bemoaning our inability to emulate and participate more actively. I maintain that vicarious participation in and through what other valued people do is an art that enhances primary morale, just as being a spectator but not a participant lifts up our spirits and makes us feel as if we belong in the company of competent, creative people. We can participate in the presence of good and skillful people who cope and create things and performances in specially gifted ways. Vicarious participation is a value in that it provides a positive experience, not one of regret. The success of others establishes continuity for us, especially with the next generation.

Every generation rues being born too soon, and mostly deplores the younger generation. When this happens, the aged are the losers. If prediction is possible, we can be quite sure that the next generation will repeat our mistakes but with their own twist. Vicarious participation would therefore mean to take a certain responsibility for a dismal legacy. This type of participation is hardly what I mean by a positive value, because it would not do much for our self-esteem. The continuity that the deserving aged yearn for is the result of having tried to count for something that would justify having lived. If this noble aim is feasible, then those who now participate vicariously would be noticed by more gifted people, appreciated for being someone who tried to preserve high standards through personal activity, not merely professing them. My image is of the actors, musicians, athletes, and artists, giving an ovation to the aged audience.

Communication between generations

Vicarious participation is not required for an older person to communicate with someone younger, but it does take considerable skill. Perhaps the chief requirement is not to think there is anything special about it but simply to admit that communication is very difficult indeed. At this moment, gazing out the window, I see birds flying from branch to branch, a squirrel scurries about, and leaves are talking to each other in a thousand, interrupting tongues. But this day is no different from any other sunny spring morning eons ago, and more recently, when Indians camped where my neighbors now live. The same day was here when I was not, longer ago than history and the ages, when my neighbors were smallish, nocturnal animals, perhaps no larger than a newt.

These very distant generations still belong to the now that I momentarily participate in. My imagined neighbors from other generations are actually no more remote or unreal than members of my own family whom I never knew, who lived just a hundred years ago. Thus, transiently, some day I shall become either totally obliterated or perhaps be a tenant on another terrain.

What then is the omega value in communication between generations? Maybe this moment is ample enough. But for the aged, its unique value might consist of finding a response, perhaps even an echo in succeeding generations, as well as in the past.

The phrase "communication between generations" sounds very majestic, but its omega value depends on calm acceptance of transience, as one generation melts into another. This is a little different from vicarious participation, which is limited to the generations on either side of us. The aged, sharply aware of their limited imprint, are in a good position to communicate without words. All the aged ask is to be noticed by the generations coming to be. By touching the evanescence of every generation, reaching back to our very remote ancestors dwelling in a cave, and now including our own, the endurance of disappearing waves of mankind will stretch into the unforetold future.

Triumph in death

Making an authentic pronouncement about the omega value of death should not be one of grim resignation or a pious expectation of future resurrection. It is so very nice to pretend that we are merely called upon to return the gift of life. Judging by the manifold misfortunes, symbolized by the Four Horesemen and their cohorts, heaped on every generation, such a gift might be gladly relinquished. Except that rarely is it given back without a struggle. Regardless of how reluctantly we surrender the life we are, we seldom have a choice about how, when, and where we die. An appropriate death is surely possible, provided that we do not ask that it be propitious, heroic, or ideal. It is preferable to an endless existence. We know when enough is enough but usually have little to say about it.

The aged have an advantage; the contrast between living and dying, so pronounced in earlier years, has been smoothed out and cooled down. Discontinuity and separation can be dealt with. Days will succeed each other, and by so doing, given plenty of time now, ages will accumulate, and mosses will celebrate the deaths of generations yet unborn. Perhaps the supreme omega value is to arrive at a serene viewpoint in which we choose transience, just as we learn when someone we love has died that bereavement yields ultimately to the adjudication of time itself.

There is triumph in death, especially when we stop thinking that death is an inimical evil force. Death cures diseases and relieves the pain that medicine is unable to cope with. While I do not deem death my enemy, I do not, at this moment, accept its friendship. The grand strategy best suited for the journey toward limbo is to manage the prospect of extinction and transience without becoming demoralized. Death intimidates, but pious propaganda about survival in some unspecified form satirizes self-esteem.

Our obligation to cope well enough to make survival significant is about all we can be sure about. We are therefore advised to instruct ourselves in the strategies for coping better, even though we are often bewildered by cloudy conjectures about what we are coping with. In this we resemble the extinct dodo. However, if we can learn that self-instruction has no curriculum, and that omega values test us only when life cycles complete their trajectories, then coping sustains morale. The search completes itself when transience blends with a modest sense of transcendence. Then we discover a quiet triumph in being transitory.

BIBLIOGRAPHY

Adler, G., and P. Myerson, *Confrontation in Psychotherapy*. New York: Science House, 1978.

Allport, G. W. *Personality and Social Encounter: Selected Essays*. Boston: Beacon Press, 1960.

Becker, E. *The Denial of Death*. New York: The Free Press, 1973.

Bird, B. *Talking with Patients*. 2d ed. Philadelphia and Toronto: J. B. Lippincott Company, 1973.

Buie, D. *Empathy: Its Nature and Limitations*. Journal of American Psychoanal Assn. 29: 281–307, 1981.

Cassirer, E. *An Essay on Man: An Introduction to a Philosophy of Human Culture*. Garden City, NY: Doubleday, 1953.

Coelho, G., D. Hamburg, and J. Adams. eds. *Coping and Adaptation*. New York: Basic Books, 1974.

Cullen, J., B. Fox, and R. Isom, eds. *Cancer: The Behavioral Dimensions*. New York: Raven Press, 1976.

Ellenberger, H. *The Discovery of the Unconscious: The History and Evolution of Dynamic Psychiatry*. New York: Basic Books, 1970.

Erikson, E. *Childhood and Society*. New York: W. W. Norton, 1950.

Feifel, H., ed. *New Meanings of Death*. New York: McGraw-Hill (Blakiston Publication), 1977.

Frank, J. *Persuasion and Healing*. Baltimore: Johns Hopkins Press, 1961.

Frank, J. *Psychotherapy and the Human Predicament: A Psychosocial Approach*. Edited by P. Dietz. New York: Schocken Books, 1978.

Goldberger, L., and S. Breznitz, eds. *Handbook of Stress: Theoretical and Clinical Aspects*. New York: The Free Press, 1982.

Goldstein, K. *Human Nature in the Light of Psychopathology*. The William James Lectures, 1938–39. Cambridge, MA: Harvard University Press, 1940.

Haan, N. *Coping and Defending: Processes of Self-environment Organization*. New York: Academic Press, 1977.

Hillman, J. *Emotion: A Comprehensive Phenomenology of Theories and Their Meanings for Therapy*. London: Routledge and Kegan Paul, 1960.

Holland, J. "Psychologic Aspects of Cancer." In *Cancer Medicine*, edited by J. Holland and E. Frei, pp. 991–1021. Philadelphia: Lea & Febiger, 1973.

Horowitz, M. J. *Stress Response Syndromes*. New York: Jason Aronson, 1976.

James, W. *Essays on Faith and Morals*. New York: Meridian Books, New American Library, 1962.

Janis, I., and L. Mann. *Decision-making: A Psychological Analysis of Conflict, Choice and Commitment*. New York: The Free Press, 1977.

Josephson, E., and M. Josephson. *Man Alone: Alienation in Modern Society*. New York: Dell Publishing Company, 1962.

Kastenbaum, R. *Death, Society and Human Experience*. 2d ed. St. Louis: C. V. Mosby, 1981.

Kelman, H. "Kairos. The auspicious moment." *American Journal of Psychoanalysis* 29 (1969): 59–83.

Kroeber, T. C. "The Coping Functions of the Ego Mechanism."

In *The Study of Lives*, pp. 178–198. New York: Atherton Press, 1963.

Lazarus, R. *Psychological Stress and the Coping Process*. New York: McGraw-Hill, 1966.

Lewis, J. "Practicum in Attention to Affect: A course for beginning psychotherapists." *Psychiatry* 37 (1974): 109–113.

Lidz, T. "The life-cycle." In *Comprehensive Textbook of Psychiatry/III*, edited by H. Kaplan, A. Freedman, and B. Sadock, 3d ed., pp. 114–134. Baltimore: Williams & Wilkins Company, 1980.

Lipowski, Z., ed. *Advances in Psychosomatic Medicine: Psychosocial Aspects of Physical Illness*, vol. 8. London, and New York: S. Karger, 1972.

Luborsky, L., B. Singer, and L. Luborsky. "Comparative studies of psychotherapy." *Archives of General Psychiatry* 32 (1975): 995–1008.

Maslow, A. H. *The Farther Reaches of Human Nature*. New York: The Viking Press, 1971.

McCall, R. "On the Nature of Psychology: A Sceptical Clinician's view." *Journal of Clinical Psychology* 20 (1964): 311–325.

Meichenbaum, D. *Cognitive-behavior Modification*. New York: Plenum, 1977.

Menninger, K. *Man Against Himself*. New York: Harcourt Brace Jovanovich, 1938.

Moos, R., ed. *Human Adaptation: Coping with Life Crises*. Lexington, Toronto, and London: D.C. Heath, 1976.

Murphy, L., and A. Moriarity. *Vulnerability, Coping and Growth from Infancy to Adolescence*. New Haven and London: Yale University Press, 1976.

Polanyi, M. *Personal Knowledge: Toward a Post-critical Philosophy*. New York and Evanston: Harper Torch Books, 1964.

Poon, L., ed. *Aging in the Nineteen-Eighties: Psychological Issues*. New York: American Psychological Association, 1980.

Rogers, C. R. *Client-centered Therapy: Its Current Practice, Implications and Theory*. Boston and New York: Houghton Mifflin, 1951.

Schmale, A. H. "Coping Reactions of the Cancer Patient and His Family." In *Catastrophic Illness in the Seventies: Critical Issues and Complex Decisions*. New York: Proceedings of the Fourth National Symposium, Cancer Care, Inc., 1970.

Schur, M. *Freud: Living and Dying*. New York: International Universities Press, 1972.

Shneidman, E. *Deaths of Man*. New York: Quadrangle/The New York Times Book Company, 1973.

Silver, R., and C. Wortman. "Coping with Undesirable Life Events." In *Human Helplessness*, edited by J. Garber and M. Seligman, pp. 279–375. New York: Academic Press, 1980.

Sobel, D. S., ed. *Ways of Health: Holistic Approaches to Ancient and Contemporary Medicine*. New York and London: Harcourt Brace Jovanovich, 1979.

Sontag, S. *Illness as Metaphor*. New York: Farrar Straus and Giroux, 1977.

Stotland, E. *The Psychology of Hope: An Integration of Experimental Clinical and Social Approaches*. San Francisco: The Jossey-Bass Behavioral Science Series, 1969.

Sze, W., ed. *The Human Life-cycle*. New York: Jason Aronson, 1975.

Veatch, R. *Death, Dying, and the Biological Revolution: Our Last Quest for Responsibility*. New Haven and London: Yale University Press, 1976.

Weisman, A. D. *Coping with Cancer*. New York: McGraw-Hill, 1979.

————"Coping with Illness." In *Handbook of General Psychiatry*, edited by T. Hackett and N. Cassem, pp. 264–275. St. Louis: C. V. Mosby, 1978.

————*The Existential Core of Psychoanalysis: Reality Sense and Responsibility*. Boston: Little, Brown, 1965.

————"A Model for Psychosocial Phasing in Cancer." *General Hospital Psychiatry* (1979): 187–195.

————and H. R. Brettell. The Dying Patient. In *Family Practice*, 2d ed., edited by R. E. Rakel, H. F. Conn, and T. W. Johnson, pp. 249–257. Philadelphia: W. B. Saunders, 1978.

————and H. J. Sobel. "Coping with Cancer Through Self-instruction: A Hypothesis." *Journal of Human Stress* 5 (1979): 3–8.

————and J. Worden. *Coping and Vulnerability in Cancer Patients: A Research Report.* Boston: Massachusetts General Hospital, 1977.

Whitehead, A. N. *Adventures of Ideas.* New York: Macmillan, 1933.

Woodger, J. H. *Biology and Language: An Introduction to the Methodology of the Biological Sciences Including Medicine.* Cambridge, Cambridge University Press, 1952.

Wright, B. A. *Physical Disability: A Psychological Approach.* New York: Harper & Row, 1960.

Zinker, J., and S. Fink. "The Possibility for Psychological Growth in a Dying Person." *Journal of General Psychology* 74 (1966): 185–199.

INDEX

Abstinence, as coping strategy,
51–52
Acquiescence, 31, 38, 50, 56, 57
Aging, xvi, 7, 24, 112–115, 120,
130, 145
and cancer, 114
and death, 132–133
and goals, 149–150
individuality in, 148
and politico-economic power,
131–132
and psychosexuality, 123,
151–152
and solitude, 150–151
and values, 146–157
Alcohol abuse, 51, 125
Alienation, 72–73, 104, 125, 132,
150
Angst, 82–84
Annihilation, 70–71, 132
Authority, 9–12, 31
Autonomy, 9–12, 31, 32, 45
failure of, 102
and pain, 26

Blame, as coping strategy, 57–58,
60, 98, 154

Cancer, xiii, 48–49
and authority vs. autonomy, 11
mortality, 15, 19, 29, 30, 71, 114

as myth, xiii, 15–17
and prejudice, 17
and psychiatric illness, 86, 87
and psychotherapy, 85–90
treatment of, 85
victims of, 17
Care givers, 81
and cancer patients, 86–92
see also Psychotherapy
Chronology, 117–118, 127
Coexistence, 142–145
vs. competition, 143–144
Communication, 65, 67, 81, 126
between generations, 155–156
Conformity, as coping strategy,
55–57
Confrontation, as coping strategy,
45–47, 64
Consolation, 38, 56
Criminality, 56, 57

Death, xii–xiii, xiv, 14, 16, 25, 33,
153, 156–157
appropriate, 80–82, 132, 157
and deathliness, 28–30
fear of, 77, 79
postponement of, xii, 34, 132
realization of, 132–133
responses to, 102
Demoralization, 27–28
vocational, 97–98
Denial, 60–62, 74–76
and illusion, 80

Depression, 69
Developmental interactions,
     118–119
Disability, 26–27, 113
Disposition, 68, 70
Distraction, as coping strategy,
     44–45
Dodo, 138–141, 143, 145, 157
Dysphoria, 25–26, 40, 41, 42,
     68–69, 81
   and vulnerability, 68

Education, 7–8
Embarrassment, 68
Emotional release, 59–60
Emotional tone, 40–42
Empathy, 105–106, 125
Endangerment, 73–74
Escape, as coping strategy, 54–55
Existentialism, xiv, xv, 40, 52, 59,
     69
   and alienation, 72–73
   and annihilation, 70–71
   in cancer, 86, 89–90
   and death, 102
   and denial, 74–76
   and endangerment, 73–74
   and illusion, 80

Forgiveness, 58
   in old age, 153

Grief, 68
Guilt, 8, 59

Health, 21, 119–120
Holistic medicine, 119–120
Hypervigilance, as coping
     strategy, 43

Ideological affiliations, 126–127
Illness, 13, 14, 15, 17, 21–22, 29,
     38, 120
Illusion, 76–82
Information, as coping strategy,
     37–38, 56, 65
Intermediate strategies, 136–138

Laughter, as coping strategy
     40–42
Life cycles, xv, 112–133, 134,
     142, 146, 157

Meaning, 2, 30, 32, 33, 34, 66–69,
     71–72, 77
Metaproblems, 30, 53
Morale, 12, 30, 33, 34, 63–64, 79,
     157
   in cancer, 91
   and death, 80, 81
   mutual, 142
   primary, 83, 136, 155
   in psychotherapists, 98
   secondary, 84, 137
Mortality; see Cancer; Death
Myths, xiii, 2, 15, 140
   and disease, 15–19

Negation; see Denial

Omega values, 146–157

Pain, 26, 106, 153, 157
Personal style, 129–130
Politico-economic deployment,
     130–132
Problems
   changing, 5, 6
   expectable, xii, xiv, 14, 19–30,
     124, 133, 146

financial, 20–21
  as metaproblems, 30, 33–34
  and survival, 23, 35
Psychosexual fulfillment, 122–123
Psychosocial adaptation, 121–122
Psychotherapy, 8, 27, 85–111

Redefinition, as coping strategy,
  47–49, 130
Reflection
  as coping strategy, 53–54
  in old age, 149
Repetition compulsion, 6
Resignation, as coping strategy,
  49–50

Self-instruction, 4–9, 11–12, 34,
  37–38, 45, 55, 61, 62, 107,
  149, 157

Skepticism, 7, 110, 136
Suicide, 14, 27, 52, 64
Suppression, as coping strategy,
  42–43

Thanatologic realization, 132–133
Thanatology, xii, 79

Unemployment, 33
  as metaphor for disease, 21

Vulnerability, 63–64, 66, 83–84,
  104
  and aging, 146

Work ethic, exemption from,
  147–148
Worry, as coping strategy, 42–43,
  44